Heal Your Headache

Heal Your Headache

The 1-2-3 Program for
Taking Charge of Your Pain

———————

DAVID BUCHHOLZ, M.D.

Foreword by Stephen G. Reich, M.D.

WORKMAN PUBLISHING • NEW YORK

Illustrations by Christoph Blumrich © 2002
Design by Janet Parker

Cataloging and publication information is available
from the Library of Congress.
ISBN 0-7611-2798-4 (hc)
ISBN 07611-2566-3 (paper)

Workman books are available at special discounts when purchased
in bulk for premiums and sales promotions as well as for fund-raising
or educational use.

Special editions or book excerpts can be created to specification.
For details, contact the Special Sales Director at the address below.

Workman Publishing Company, Inc.
708 Broadway
New York, NY 10003-9555
www.workman.com

Printed in the United States of America
First printing: August 2002
10 9 8 7 6 5 4 3 2 1

To my patients, who taught me about headaches

Acknowledgments

WHEN I GRADUATED from high school in 1970, I was a lost soul. The only thing I knew for sure was that I didn't want to go to college. I dreamed of writing a book but didn't have anything to say. Harold Kundel, a radiology researcher at Temple University, took me under his wing as a lab assistant for three years. With his help I grew up a lot, eventually going to college and beyond. I shudder to think where I would have wound up without him; yet until now I've never really said thanks.

During my college years Martin Seligman, a professor at the University of Pennsylvania, encouraged me to go to graduate school in psychology rather than medical school, but I leaned the other way. His argument was that as a medical doctor I might directly care for as many as tens of thousands of patients over the years, but as a research psychologist I could make a discovery that could catch on and benefit vastly more people. I didn't follow his advice, but I never lost sight of his challenge, and I smile to think how great it would be if it turned out, after all, that this book might have such impact.

After I completed my neurology training at Johns Hopkins, Guy McKhann, the department chair, welcomed me to the faculty even though I was strictly a clinician, a people doctor, and not (as is generally the rule at Hopkins) also a researcher. In that position I met my many headache patients and gained the special experience from which grew the understanding of headaches that lies at the heart of this book. Thanks also to Chip Moses, who I suspect twisted Guy's arm.

In 1991 the Johns Hopkins University Press sent me a headache manuscript for review. I panned it ("the same old stuff") and suggested I could do better. Jackie Wehmueller, the acquiring editor, offered me the opportunity to put my money where my mouth was. It took me more than seven years to get around to a first draft, but Jackie's been a devoted proponent every halting step and misstep along the way. Without her, I'm not sure that this book would ever have materialized.

Two other people played vital roles in the development of this book. For years I worked side by side at Hopkins with Stephen Reich, and together we tackled the problem of migraine, me pushing the envelope and he reining me in with much-needed reality checks. And then there was Charles Wasserman, who helped me overcome—even if not understand—the forces that had held me back from writing all those years.

Scott Sherman, then a dean at the medical school, contributed by making sure that my first draft found its way into the right hands. Through him I eventually contacted Channa Taub, my agent, who understood that it was critical for me to write the book myself, in my own words, rather than with a ghostwriter. It was also through Scott that I connected with Susan Bolotin, editor-in-chief at Workman, who shepherded the project into print and showed me that skillful editing is the greatest gift a writer can receive.

Harold Nussenfeld and Christian van den Bos provided helpful feedback along the way. Michael Kandel was always there with his strong support and faithful friendship. And my extraordinarily competent, dedicated and tolerant secretary, Carolyn McCormack, managed to juggle this project along with her usual three handfuls of other work, all with a smile on her face, laughter in her voice and kindness in her heart. Thank you all.

Steffi Neumann, my wife, paid a dear price in putting up—night after night and year after year—with my endless musings and rantings about the book. More substantially, she is responsible for most of the Appendix. (Try the recipes; she's a wonderful cook.) And more importantly, the love and friendship we share has sustained me at times when this book felt more like an ordeal than an accomplishment.

Too often, my work has kept me from my children, Brittany, Alison and Max. I thank them for their patience and for believing in me as much as I believe in them.

Finally, I thank my parents. I know you're proud, and that makes me happy.

Contents

Foreword

DURING THE LAST 20 YEARS, David Buchholz has helped thousands of people heal their headaches. This book is the result of that experience—seeing patients with headaches day in and day out, listening carefully to them and thinking critically about what he saw. Over time, Dr. Buchholz has come to question and ultimately challenge many of the popular conventions about headache diagnosis and treatment. His hope is that this book will challenge you to think critically, too, and ultimately to think differently about headaches. If you can do that, and if you follow Dr. Buchholz's three-step approach, you will learn how to escape from living headache to headache. And you will come to realize that headache control is not only possible, but also largely in your own hands.

For over a decade, David Buchholz and I worked next door to each other in the Neurology clinic at Johns Hopkins. Hardly a day passed that we didn't discuss our most difficult and perplexing patients. I have him to thank for expanding my horizons about headaches and enabling me to help many frustrated, "failed" patients. I learned firsthand how he approached the most challenging headache sufferers. This usually began by *undoing* the many popular and well-intentioned but essentially counterproductive treatments they'd come to rely on, and then guiding patients on the right path to headache control.

A self-admitted iconoclast, Dr. Buchholz puts forth a convincing argument that migraine is far and away the most common cause of a vast array of headaches and other related symptoms. Why is that important? Because once you understand the mechanism of migraine, you will realize how to control it and prevent its symptoms.

You're wondering, *What magic does Dr. Buchholz have?* His answer, perhaps surprisingly, would be, *None*. Instead, the effectiveness of the 1-2-3 Program outlined in this book lies in its simplicity and in its conviction that *you* have the power to make it work. Much of Dr. Buchholz's success in helping people heal their headaches is his ability to communicate effectively and persuasively, as he does so clearly here. And as you'll see, his advice is not just for those with severe headaches, but for all those who seek to rid themselves of every form of head discomfort.

This thoughtful and provocative book will show you how, in three steps, to transform yourself from feeling a helpless victim of headaches to being in control of them.

Stephen G. Reich, M.D.
Department of Neurology
University of Maryland School of Medicine
Baltimore, Maryland

Introduction

THIS BOOK IS ABOUT MIGRAINE, which is not whatever you think it is. It's much, much more. It's within you—yes, *you*—and all around you.

In part this book is about headaches—what causes them and how you can control them. But you'll also learn the real story behind dizziness, neck stiffness, sinus congestion and other common disturbances that invade our lives. Together, we'll explore dark corners of human nature into which we're led by following paths of least resistance and where we become trapped in cycles of victimization and dependence, blame and guilt. If you're stuck in such a corner, I can show you the way out.

Ultimately this book is about control—how you lose it and how to regain it. If you really want to control your headaches and other migraine symptoms, I can help you. Headaches are *natural*, but they're not *necessary*. By doing the right things, you can transform your life. Follow me: I'll teach you how to take charge of your headaches.

The Truth About Headaches

IF YOU'RE LIKE MOST PEOPLE, you're probably confused about the whole subject of headaches. You may wonder, Do I have migraine? (And what *is* migraine, anyway?) Or do I have a brain tumor? Could it be an aneurysm? What about my tension headaches? Or sinus headaches? Is it arthritis in my neck, or a pinched nerve, or am I just stressed out, or is it my hormones, or . . . *what is it?*

Maybe you're frustrated, too, because your headaches aren't under control. Painkillers help temporarily (sometimes, at least), but you're not sure when your next headache will strike or whether the quick fix will work. (And *God forbid* it should run out!) You may also have nagging stiffness in your neck or congestion in your sinuses that never lets up.

You're not the only one who's confused and frustrated about headaches. Odds are, so are your family, your friends and your doctor. If your doctor has prescribed painkillers but you're still struggling with headaches, you're probably feeling frustrated with each other. No wonder. You and your doctor are dealing with headaches the wrong way.

The right way begins with the knowledge that nearly all headaches, of all types, arise from a single mechanism—the mechanism of migraine—that is built into us by nature and generates painful blood vessel swelling when activated by specific triggers. This headache-generating mechanism, which produces not only headaches but also other symptoms including dizziness, neck stiffness, sinus congestion and many more, can be controlled. Control starts with reducing your exposure to some of its triggers, especially certain foods and medications. If trigger avoidance alone isn't effective, preventive medication, which blocks the mechanism, can be added. Painkillers, on the other hand, lead you to lose control. Many headache sufferers spin farther and farther out of control in a vicious cycle of victimization by headaches and dependence on painkillers.

Conventional medical wisdom mistakenly divides headaches into innumerable types, relegating the diagnosis of migraine to a small fraction—the extreme end—of its true spectrum. When fully activated, the mechanism of migraine generates full-blown episodes of severe, stereotyped headaches with nausea and visual disturbances that are recognized as "migraines." But far more frequently we experience mild-to-moderate, nonspecific headaches, neck discomfort and sinus congestion—not to mention dizziness and much more—arising from *partial* activation of the mechanism. Routinely, these symptoms are misdiagnosed as tension headache, sinus headache or something else other than migraine. Misdiagnosis leads to mistreatment, which leads to failure, confusion and frustration. Sound familiar?

Even when migraine *is* diagnosed, too many headache sufferers and their doctors rely on the quick-fix approach of painkillers. In other words, instead of taking control of your headaches, you're on the run from them; you're a victim, reacting defensively. As you become more and more dependent on painkillers, and as these drugs become less and less effective, the quick-fix approach creates rebound: a state of never-ending headaches (and inability to respond to preventive treatment that would otherwise control them).

And so, relying on painkillers, headache sufferers find themselves getting worse instead of better. But with the right approach to diagnosis and treatment, headaches (and the other symptoms of migraine) can be *controlled*. You can accomplish this by following the 1-2-3 Program set forth in this book.

Blaming the Patient

WHEN I FINISHED my neurology training 20 years ago, I thought I knew all about headaches. Mostly I knew that I didn't like seeing headache patients. Too often, they didn't get better, and frankly I considered them to be a nuisance. Looking back I see why—and why I was so wrong. Caring for headache patients *can* be a nuisance when your approach to diagnosing and treating headaches is wrong, as is the conventional approach I learned (and, probably, so did your doctor) in medical school. Patients don't get better when they're diagnosed and treated incorrectly, and when patients don't get better, it's frustrating.

To account for headache treatment failure, doctors have two options: (1) question conventional wisdom, or (2) blame the patient. And not surprisingly, it's the second option that wins out. Blaming the patient takes many forms. Sometimes headache patients are labeled whiners, gripers, complainers or drug-seekers. Often chronic headache sufferers are assumed to be neurotic or depressed. Doctors may insinuate that, given your load of personal problems (work, marriage, family, financial), it's *inevitable* that you suffer from headaches. Or the implicit message is: *Your headaches are all in your head.* One way or the other, it's your fault. Either you like to complain, or you're after something (such as painkillers), or you're a sorry person, or you deserve your headaches, or you just imagine them.

Whatever form it takes, blaming headache patients for treatment failure is a triple-play opportunity for doctors. In one fell swoop, doctors can (1) wash their hands of personal responsibility, (2) instead, displace potential guilt onto patients, and (3) safely avoid questioning conventional wisdom. Thus conventional wisdom about headaches has a built-in defense mechanism to assure its survival. It *predicts* that many headache patients who are diagnosed and treated "by the book" will fail, not through any fault of its own but because of faults of *their* own: *Of course headache patients fail! What do you expect? They're headache patients!* More than just a self-serving attitude, this becomes a self-fulfilling prophecy.

Now let's consider this situation from the patient's perspective. The resistant patient who hesitates to accept blame and bear guilt for persistent headaches is all the more likely to be labeled a "problem" patient. Complaining not only about headaches but also about failure of treatment fortifies the doctor's suspicion that you're someone who just likes to complain. Many headache patients don't resist accepting blame for treatment failure; they swallow it whole. Whether they're blamed explicitly or implicitly, who are they to question a *doctor's* judgment of their guilt? (Family, friends and coworkers conspire unwittingly by questioning the validity of chronic headache complaints: *How can anyone have a headache every day?*)

Blame for treatment failure does not belong primarily to headache patients; more often their doctors are responsible. Maybe doctors *do* sense this at some level, and maybe that's in part why—truth be told, whether they can or will admit it—most doctors don't like to see headache patients.

A few years back I was about to give a lecture entitled *Top 10 Reasons Why Your Headache Patients Don't Get Better* and was having second thoughts about my closing slide, which read: "Reason #1— You Don't Like Headache Patients." I was afraid it might be a bit rude, but just before my lecture I bumped into the neurologist who organized the symposium. I asked who was in the audience, and he mentioned doctors from various specialties and added, "Some of the pain weasels have come out, too." The pain weasels were his headache patients. My second thoughts about the slide vanished. He, not I, was the rude one.

And so I became even more determined not to pull any punches in my assault on the ignorance and attitudes within my profession that have caused so many headache sufferers to suffer needlessly. Some colleagues may accuse me of doctor-bashing and being disloyal. Well, my loyalty is to headache sufferers. And here's what I have to say to those who would argue that I'm undermining people's faith in their doctors: *I would* hope *I am*, if *that faith is blind, misplaced and counterproductive.*

I think there are two reasons why I've not only been able to look at migraine in a different way but also am willing to spread the word about it. The first is the unique experience I've had at Johns Hopkins, where for 20 years my particular role has been as a go-to guy for patients with neurological problems whose symptoms defied explanation (despite numerous, thorough prior evaluations) and who failed to respond to multiple (misguided) treatment approaches. There are basically three possible explanations for the difficulties these many people face: (1) they might have a variety of elusive, esoteric diseases; (2) they might suffer from any number of psychological or emotional conditions masquerading as physical illness; or (3) they might be experiencing something fairly *common* that has escaped recognition because no one has looked at it the right way. And that, as it turns out, is so often the case. It's migraine. From seeing hundreds upon hundreds of patients with no reasonable explanation for their complaints other than "atypical" migraine, it began to dawn on me that simply *migraine*, much more broadly defined, was the culprit.

The other source of my ability to not only see but also speak the truth about migraine is more personal; it has to do with my inclination to be an ornery instigator. I'm naturally contrarian, and I don't mind messing with orthodoxy. Frankly, I *like* to make trouble for the establishment when it's at fault, and if doing so helps people solve their problems. As much as some may see me *only* as a troublemaker, I see myself—and hope you'll see me—as a problem-solver when it comes to your headaches and other bothersome migraine symptoms.

The Tough-Love Approach

THE CORRECT APPROACH to headaches is simple—though not necessarily easy. It's an approach that discourages quick fixes and emphasizes durable self-control of your headaches. You must accept responsibility for your headaches and exert your will to control them. As explained in this book, the 1-2-3 Program to control your headaches *works* and is gratifying for headache sufferers, their doctors and everyone else involved. For me, learning the right approach to headaches—in effect, becoming Dr. Tough Love—is how I learned to stop worrying and love headache patients . . . or at least love helping them control their headaches.

You may wonder whether I myself have ever suffered from headaches. The answer is, I used to get a fair number of moderate headaches (and a memorable doozy once in a blue moon). And after years of advising my patients to avoid certain dietary triggers, it gradually dawned on me that my headaches, like theirs, were being fed by what I was eating and drinking. I became more careful about these items, and now I have only rare, mild headaches. The point is, I never was a big-time headache sufferer. So does this mean I can't help you because I can't "feel your pain"? No, to the contrary, I think I can help you all the better. It's hard enough for me to stand firm and refuse to cave in to pleas for quick fixes from acutely suffering patients. If I related more strongly to their desperation from extensive personal experience, I don't know if I could keep doing the right thing: standing firm and guiding them from the morass. And I don't know if I'd be able to do the same for you.

The 1-2-3 Program Works

THIS BOOK IS NOT JUST for those who have struggled with the extremes of migraine pain for years. It can help you even if you suffer from headaches only occasionally. Do you experience "sinus" headaches when the weather changes or "tension" headaches with stress? Is your neck often stiff, or are you frequently congested? Maybe your child has complained that his head hurts in school, and you haven't known what to do. Does your teenager have headaches with her periods, month after month? And how about your friend who gets dizzy spells? (Or is it *you* who's dizzy all the time?)

The foundation of the 1-2-3 Program is a clear understanding of the migraine mechanism and the broad spectrum of headaches and other symptoms it generates. Once you've read all the chapters in this book, you'll be prepared to take the right steps to prevent its activation—and thereby prevent the symptoms that result. *Step 1* puts painkillers in their proper place: infrequent use only. Quick fixes for headaches aren't your friends; if anything, they're the enemy. They cause you to lose control, and you won't get it back until you achieve independence from them. *Step 2* is eliminating headache triggers that you can readily control—mainly those that you put in your mouth and swallow. If you can keep your total trigger level below your threshold for activation of migraine, the mechanism will not become activated and you'll be symptom-free.

If you respond well enough to the first two steps, *Step 3* may not be needed. If it does prove necessary, preventive medication (taken on a daily basis) can be added to block activation of migraine and thereby prevent the headaches and other symptoms it generates. Used properly, one or more of several preventive medication options can safely and effectively control your headaches.

But before we begin, let's be clear about a few things. Most of the ideas expressed in this book did not originate with me. Many other headache specialists, past and present, have contributed to the understanding of headaches that I'm about to lay out for you. My contribution is to take some of these ideas a step further, blend the correct mix and present it so that it makes perfect sense. What I offer is a conceptual model of migraine, based in part on scientific data generated by others and in part on my own experience successfully helping thousands of patients to control their headaches over a period of two decades.

In scientific terms, my beliefs are hypotheses: potential explanations of certain cause-and-effect relationships. In this case, the migraine mechanism is one cause. When activated by sufficient triggers, the effects produced by this mechanism include all types of headaches and a host of other symptoms. Another cause is rebound, which results from dependence on quick-fix painkillers. Its effects are increased headaches and resistance to preventive treatment of migraine.

Scientists may wish to test these hypotheses formally, using randomized controlled trials. Memo to colleagues who undertake this challenge: Good luck, and I hope you do it right. *If* that's possible. Helping people control their headaches by guiding them to do the right things demands art, and science in the form of a clinical trial might just interfere. Simply telling people *what* to do—without adequately explaining *why*, without forcefully countering resistance to what people don't want to hear and without offering confident, optimistic encouragement—*won't* work. Don't forget: the process of science inevitably disturbs whatever it studies and therefore never really studies what it means to.

And setting aside the 20 years it's taken me to refine my skills in teaching people to control their headaches, I know that my passionate faith in the 1-2-3 Program could not possibly be possessed, let alone conveyed, by dispassionate investigators conducting a controlled trial of my approach. I would not even participate in such a trial, because I *know* that the 1-2-3 Program works and I would not want any patient of mine to be randomized to alternative (and less effective) "control" treatment.

The final and most important hypothesis I offer is that by dealing properly with migraine and rebound you can control their effects: the headaches and other symptoms that result. In my extensive experience with headache patients, this hypothesis has been put to the test repeatedly and has passed time and again. The test is: by using the 1-2-3 Program, can headaches and other symptoms of migraine be controlled? Emphatically, the answer is *yes*. No "scientific" data to the contrary, from a randomized controlled trial or any other source, would ever convince me otherwise.

Don't get me wrong: science *can* be a valuable tool. But sometimes you can recognize truth on your own, without needing scientists to certify it for you, because when you open your eyes and look at things the right way, the truth becomes obvious. Decide for yourself whether or not what I have to say rings true—in fact, *makes perfect sense*.

The details of my model of migraine may not be completely accurate—after all, the details remain largely unknown to anyone—but for our purposes that's not so important. What *is* important is that this model is *effective* in guiding you to control your headaches. It provides a framework that helps you understand *why* you have to do *what* you have to do. With faith in yourself and a clear plan—the 1-2-3 Program—you *can* control your headaches.

THE TRUTH
ABOUT MIGRAINE

CHAPTER ONE

What Is Migraine?

E veryone gets headaches. About 90 percent of people surveyed *admit* to having them; the other 10 percent either (a) simply wouldn't *call* their discomfort a headache, (b) have headaches too mild or infrequent to remember, (c) experience headaches with hangovers and would just as soon forget them, (d) are having a good day when asked, (e) are stubborn, (f) are in denial, or (g) don't understand the question.

We all get headaches because nature has built into us a headache-generating mechanism. This mechanism, called migraine, has the potential to produce swelling and inflammation of blood vessels around your head. It is a universal mechanism—*everyone has it*—but it varies individually in its levels of activation and forms of expression.

When *fully* activated, the mechanism of migraine produces severe head pain, commonly accompanied by nausea, vomiting, sensitivity to bright light (photophobia) and loud noise (phonophobia), and sometimes visual disturbances and other neurological symptoms. When *partially* activated, as is much more often the case, this same mechanism results in mild-to-moderate, nonspecific discomfort in or around your head, face or neck and is much less likely to be accompanied by the kinds of other symptoms that are thought to characterize migraine.

It's a mistake to think of one particular type of headache as "a migraine," since the migraine mechanism can generate *any* kind of headache. Moreover, as discussed later on, this mechanism can cause many other symptoms, *with or without* headache.

Where It All Begins

SOMEWHERE IN THE BRAIN lies the migraine control center, which receives the flow of triggers that activate the mechanism. Where this center is located, no one knows for sure, but the hypothalamus is the most obvious candidate. This deep-seated part of the brain controls many basic functions, including your sleep-wake cycle, hunger and satiety, hormonal regulation, and the autonomic (involuntary) nervous system.

Several features of the hypothalamus make it the most likely site of the migraine control center. To start with, virtually all migraine activators have input to the hypothalamus (see Figure 1, page 5). For instance, emotional triggers such as stress (or letdown after stress) and depression involve the brain's limbic system, of which the hypothalamus is a part. In addition, hormonal triggers such as estrogen are regulated by the hypothalamus and have special access to it. (In order to be able to monitor hormones, the hypothalamus lacks the normal blood-brain barrier that shields most of the brain from substances circulating in the bloodstream.)

Chemical triggers in foods and beverages can also reach the hypothalamus as they circulate in the bloodstream following absorption from the gut. Migraine can be triggered by skipping meals as well, perhaps because of the role of the hypothalamus in overseeing hunger and

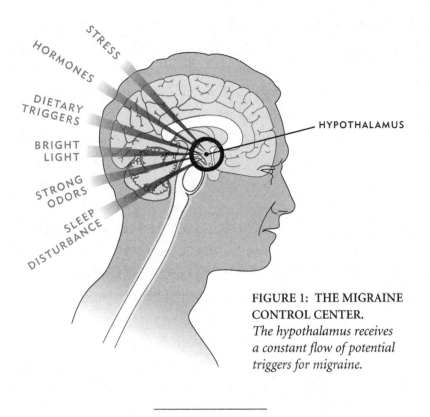

STRESS

HORMONES

DIETARY TRIGGERS

BRIGHT LIGHT

STRONG ODORS

SLEEP DISTURBANCE

HYPOTHALAMUS

FIGURE 1: THE MIGRAINE CONTROL CENTER.
The hypothalamus receives a constant flow of potential triggers for migraine.

satiety. Sensory triggers, both visual (sunlight glare, strobe lights) and olfactory (perfumes, cigarette smoke), can also reach the hypothalamus via direct nerve pathways leading from receptors in the eyes and nose.

An association between the migraine control center and the hypothalamus is likely for other reasons. Migraine is often linked to the sleep-wake cycle, which is governed by the brain's master clock, located in the hypothalamus. The relationship of migraine to the sleep-wake cycle is evident not only from fluctuations in migraine activity occurring at regular times (for instance, headaches upon awakening) but also from the triggering of migraine as a result of either sleep deprivation *or* oversleep (as on weekend mornings), as well as relief of migraine following sleep.

Are You Alone?

While many headache-prone people regard themselves as part of a long-standing family tradition, others wonder why they alone have been so unlucky. To their knowledge, no one else in the family has much of a headache problem.

Usually they're wrong. Given the many ways in which overt headache sufferers are belittled by those who don't understand, family members may choose to suffer in relative silence, even among their kin. Or a person with recognized "migraine" might not see the family connection with others' "sick," "sinus," "stress" or menstrual headaches. Acorns don't fall far from the tree, and if you look carefully for migraine—with a broad perspective in mind—you can almost always find it rooted nearby. ◆

In addition, migraine often occurs with accompanying symptoms such as nausea, vomiting, constipation, diarrhea, flushing or pallor of the skin, sweating, chills and fever—all of which reflect disturbances of the auto-nomic (involuntary) nervous system, which is governed in part by the hypothalamus.

Trigger Level vs. Threshold

TWO FACTORS DETERMINE whether or not the migraine mechanism is activated—and if so, to what degree. Understanding these two deter-minants and how they relate to each other is the key to controlling your headaches.

The first determinant of migraine activity is the *trigger level*. Triggers vary from individual to individual—what is a trigger for you might not be for me—and the total level of triggers varies in each of us from moment to moment.

The second determinant of migraine is the *threshold*: a preset level of trigger input at which the mechanism will become activated. This threshold also differs from person to person and is largely genetically determined. If you suffer from frequent, severe headaches, you likely come from a family that includes other headache sufferers. On a hereditary basis, you and your relatives have low thresholds and are therefore especially susceptible to headaches and other symptoms of migraine.

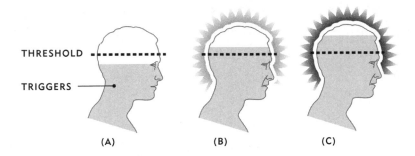

THRESHOLD

TRIGGERS

(A)   (B)   (C)

FIGURE 2: CROSSING THE THRESHOLD. *Triggers enter the migraine control center in a constant flow, activating the mechanism only when they build to a level above your threshold. As shown above, a below-threshold trigger level (A) produces no symptoms. As the trigger level rises above your threshold (B), migraine symptoms appear. As the level climbs even higher (C), symptoms increase.*

Most people—the majority who do not identify themselves as having major headache problems—have higher thresholds and therefore fewer and milder headaches.

As the total trigger level rises above the threshold, the migraine mechanism becomes activated. Generally speaking, the higher the above-threshold trigger level, the more fully activated the mechanism and the greater the symptoms (see Figure 2, above). (There's a ceiling to this, so that at *some* level the mechanism is as fully activated as it can be.) Once triggered, the mechanism can remain active for periods as short as split seconds or as long as a matter of days, even after the trigger level has fallen back below the threshold. But there may be persistent migraine activity (such as chronic daily headache or constant dizziness), lasting weeks, months or *years*, as long as the trigger level stays above the threshold.

The total level of triggers varies constantly. Dietary items, stress, medications, hormones, sensory stimuli, barometric pressure changes, sleep deprivation and other triggers add up in the control center. As you read this, you carry a stack of triggers that reflects your exposure to these influences over the past day or two. If the *sum* of your triggers exceeds your threshold, migraine becomes activated and you'll have symptoms. One day, if your trigger level is far below threshold to begin with, you might be able to eat as much chocolate as you like and get away with it. A few days later, if the barometric pressure is falling, or you're seated next to someone wearing heavy perfume, or you've been up half the night, or you're on the verge of your menstrual period, you eat just one little chocolate-chip cookie, cross the threshold and wind up with a splitting headache. The greater your trigger load, the more likely you'll get a headache and the worse it will be.

The key to controlling your headaches and other migraine symptoms is simple: *Keep your trigger level below your threshold.* This means reducing your trigger exposure, raising your threshold, or taking both steps together. By doing so, you can prevent activation of migraine and its consequences.

How Does Migraine Cause Pain?

ONCE YOUR TRIGGER LEVEL crosses your threshold and migraine becomes activated, the mechanism spreads through various parts of the brain, involving a number of neurotransmitters (chemical messengers) along the way. One of the most important neurotransmitters of migraine is serotonin, but to think of migraine as simply an imbalance of serotonin is to overlook the involvement of other neurotransmitters such as dopamine and neuropeptides. The brain is not just a chemical soup in which too much or too little of one ingredient can lead to problems. It's more like a computer, wired with many complicated circuits along which neurotransmitters relay impulses. Migraine involves one such circuit, with multiple inputs (triggers) feeding into it and outputs (symptoms) arising from it. We understand only sketchy details of this mechanism, but one thing is clear: *it can be controlled by the 1-2-3 Program.*

As migraine proceeds, a group of nerve cells in the brain stem (the trigeminal nucleus caudalis) becomes activated. Signals travel from this region along the trigeminal and upper cervical nerves to blood vessels around your head, face and neck (see Figure 3, pages 10–11). (Each of these nerves supplies one side only, which is why migraine pain can be one-sided if it stems from that pathway alone.) At this point the mechanism of migraine, which is controlled *within* the brain, has spread *outside* the brain.

Impulses traveling down these nerve fibers lead to the release of neuropeptides from nerve endings. These neurotransmitters cause blood vessels around your head to become swollen and inflamed. Nitric oxide, a chemical that produces vasodilation (blood vessel swelling), also plays a role. The resulting swelling and inflammation of blood vessels around your head generates headache (or some other form of discomfort in or around your head, face or neck).

How do blood vessel swelling and inflammation translate into the pain that you feel? Again nerve fibers play a role, but in this case the fibers carry impulses in the opposite direction: back to the brain. The swollen, inflamed blood vessels stimulate pain receptors on nerve endings, and the resulting pain signals are carried back to the brain by nerve fibers. In other words, nerves around your head are two-way streets carrying migraine traffic from and to the brain: outgoing impulses that cause swelling and inflammation of blood vessels around your head, and incoming signals reflecting the presence of blood vessel swelling and inflammation. Ultimately, when this reverberating loop becomes activated, the information that blood vessels are swollen and inflamed reaches the brain stem and is relayed to higher centers in the brain, where it is translated into the discomfort, distress and distraction that you know as a headache.

Normally, transmission of pain impulses and the experience of pain is subdued by naturally occurring, narcotic-like substances known as endogenous opioids (or endorphins). To make matters worse, the migraine mechanism somehow interferes with the endogenous opioid

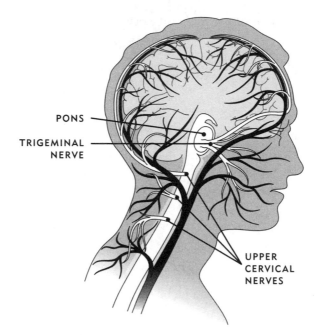

PONS

TRIGEMINAL
NERVE

UPPER
CERVICAL
NERVES

FIGURE 3: THE MIGRAINE MECHANISM. *When migraine activates, signals travel via the trigeminal and upper cervical nerves to blood vessels around your head, face and neck (depicted in black).*

---

system so that, in effect, the experience of pain generated by migraine is magnified instead of muted. Migraine makes your brain act and feel *sensitive*. Even background sensations such as pulsation of blood vessels, which are normally filtered from awareness, are instead felt as throbbing, pounding pain.

The Non-Headache Symptoms of Migraine

WE'VE SEEN HOW blood vessel swelling causes the pain of migraine, but what about its other symptoms? The *autonomic* symptoms—nausea, vomiting, constipation, diarrhea, flushing or pallor of the skin, sweating, chills and

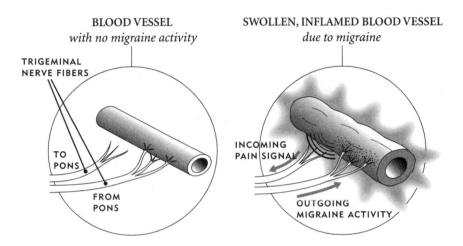

BLOOD VESSEL
with no migraine activity

SWOLLEN, INFLAMED BLOOD VESSEL
due to migraine

TRIGEMINAL
NERVE FIBERS

TO
PONS

FROM
PONS

INCOMING
PAIN SIGNAL

OUTGOING
MIGRAINE ACTIVITY

*As a result, the blood vessels swell and become inflamed, and pain
receptors on nearby nerve endings are stimulated. These nerves transmit
pain signals back to the brain, and you experience the pain of migraine.*

fever—stem from dysfunction of the part of the hypothalamus that normally governs the autonomic nervous system in an orderly fashion but misbehaves in the course of migraine. Photophobia, phonophobia and neck stiffness, all common features of migraine, arise from inflammation of blood vessels in the membranes called meninges that line the brain.

The final part of the mechanism of migraine is the most controversial. This is the part that generates *neurological* symptoms including flashing lights and other visual disturbances, dizziness, numbness and tingling. There are two rival hypotheses concerning the origin of these symptoms.

The first hypothesis contends that the neurological symptoms of migraine result from constriction of blood vessels in the brain, eye or

The One-Two Punch of Migraine

Blood vessel swelling and inflammation outside the brain cause *pain* around the head, face or neck, whereas blood vessel constriction within the brain, eye or inner ear causes the *neurological symptoms* of migraine. Migraine thereby generates two different forms of blood vessel misbehavior, and these can occur either alone or in concert. As the mechanism of migraine unfolds, it reaches a fork in the road and can travel down one path (to headache), the other path (to neurological symptoms), or both, either simultaneously or sequentially. ◆

inner ear. Transient, reversible constriction of blood vessels can take place because of the presence of muscle fibers in the walls of blood vessels. When these muscle fibers contract, blood vessels constrict. Conversely, when the muscle fibers relax, blood vessels dilate.

According to this hypothesis, temporary constriction of blood vessels in various parts of the brain, eye and inner ear results in decreased blood flow, leading to temporary dysfunction of the involved areas. The site of decreased blood flow determines the neurological symptoms that consequently occur. Involvement either of the occipital lobes of the brain, where vision is produced, or of the eye produces flashing lights or other visual disturbances. Involvement of the balance system in the brain or the inner ear causes dizziness, and involvement of somatosensory pathways leads to numbness and tingling. (As discussed in the next chapter, there's *much* more to this story.)

The second (and more recent) hypothesis holds that neurological symptoms of migraine arise primarily from electrical disturbances of brain cells. According to this hypothesis, blood vessel constriction occurs secondarily, in response to these disturbances.

Debate continues over these two hypotheses. What we do know is: (a) the mechanism of migraine is *neurovascular,* involving both nerve cells and blood vessels, (b) migraine has independent pathways that lead to pain and to neurological symptoms, (c) the pathway that leads to pain does so by causing blood vessels around your head (and face and neck) to become swollen and inflamed, and (d) the pathway leading to neurological symptoms somehow involves constriction of blood vessels in the brain, eye and inner ear.

More important than who's right about exactly what happens when migraine becomes activated is the fact that *you* can keep it from happening by following the 1-2-3 Program.

"It feels like Novocain wearing off"

JIM'S STORY

When he was a teenager, Jim had severe headaches accompanied by vomiting and sometimes preceded by his vision "fragmenting into pieces" for 10 to 20 minutes. These episodes were recognized as "migraines," and after a few years they went away.

From time to time Jim would get a "regular" headache, especially when he was under stress or didn't get enough sleep, but these were "no big deal." What brought him to see me was something altogether different. For three months, about twice a day, he'd been getting the feeling of "Novocain wearing off" on the right side of his face, lasting a matter of minutes. He feared stroke, or multiple sclerosis, or some other grave ailment.

It was just migraine. Jim followed the migraine-preventive diet I gave him and felt much better, with only a few recurrent "Novocain" episodes that occurred after eating in certain restaurants. His regular headaches disappeared—along with the extra 15 pounds he'd been carrying around! ◆

CHAPTER TWO

The Full Spectrum of Migraine

N ow that you know what migraine *is*, let's take a closer look at what it *does*. In deciding whether it's worth your while to do what you can do to control your symptoms of migraine, you'll decide more wisely if you better understand your *total burden* of migraine. It may be far heavier than you realize, and you'll be more motivated to do the right things to reduce it when you appreciate its full weight on your shoulders.

The Spectrum of Migraine Headache

NOT ONLY IS THE TERM "MIGRAINE" misleading when it's used to designate one specific type of headache, but even the term "headache" is inadequate to cover the full spectrum of discomfort generated by the migraine mechanism. Discomfort may be felt anywhere in or around the face or neck as well as the head. Words such as "ache" and "pain" may not even begin to capture the discomfort you feel as a result of migraine.

Instead, in or around your head you may experience *pressure, fullness, tightness, heaviness, thickness, numbness* or *soreness*, or you may have *swelling, burning, buzzing, vibrating, boring, piercing, drawing, expanding, tingling, trickling, bubbling, crawling, shifting* or *rushing* sensations. These sensations may be aggravated by bending over, straining, sneezing, coughing or exertion, or if you shake or jar your head.

You may have feelings suggestive more of lack of clarity than discomfort, such as *cloudiness, dullness, fogginess* or *fuzzy-headedness.* Discomfort may be excruciating, trivial or anything in between. Most of the discomfort generated by the mechanism of migraine is mild-to-moderate and nonspecific—because most often the mechanism is less than fully activated.

The severe headaches conventionally labeled "migraines" occupy a relatively narrow band at the far end of the spectrum. These headaches may be *explosive, unbearable, like a jackhammer* or *fire-hot spike.* The extreme degree of discomfort reflects the extreme degree of blood vessel swelling and inflammation when migraine is fully activated.

You may recognize that your discomfort *feels* like swollen, inflamed blood vessels around your head. For instance, migraine can generate *pulsating* and *pounding,* as if *your heart is beating in your head.* You may sense *congestion,* as you would expect with swollen blood vessels. When this occurs behind your face or in your forehead, with *stuffiness* and *postnasal drip,* you mistakenly suspect a "sinus" problem. When you have *ear fullness* with *popping* or *clicking,* you think it's an ear infection . . . when migraine is really the culprit. With swollen blood vessels throughout, your head may just feel as if *there's not enough room in there.*

You may not only feel but also *see* evidence of swollen blood vessels. Large vessels may *bulge in your temples,* or smaller vessels in the skin may dilate and cause your ear or your face to become *flushed* and

Where We Went Wrong

What led to our grossly incomplete, distorted view of migraine? It happened this way. Thousands of years ago, as today, certain individuals experienced dramatic attacks of severe, one-sided headache with vomiting. They looked like they might die. After apparently miraculous recovery within hours, these individuals said they'd seen flashing lights and other visual hallucinations. The term "migraine" (from a Greek word for half of the cranium) was coined, and it stuck. Anything apart from these dramatic episodes, including any other "type" of headache, was henceforth considered to be something other than migraine.

Only more recently was it recognized that migraine could occur without visual symptoms, and a "common" form of migraine was distinguished from the "classic" one. This recognition was but a baby step in the right direction. If you remove the blinders imposed by conventional wisdom, you can see migraine as a mechanism that's capable of producing a much, much broader spectrum of symptoms. But even when it's false, conventional wisdom remains stubborn and dies hard—because convention overrules wisdom.

When doctors diagnose migraine, it's remarkable how often they qualify their diagnosis using terms like "atypical migraine" or "migraine variant." This is understandable to a degree, because doctors who diagnose migraine when the symptoms are other than "textbook" take a risk by stepping out of the bounds of conventional wisdom. By bowing to convention and using modifiers such as "atypical" and "variant," they reduce their risk of disturbing the status quo.

Still, it's odd to describe something as atypical *so often*, without eventually questioning whether the notion of "typical" is far too restrictive. ◆

warm. Your eyes may appear *bloodshot* or *swollen,* or they may *tear. Dark circles* may form under your eyes. *Nosebleeds* can occur.

Inflammation of blood vessels around your head due to migraine causes *tenderness.* Your scalp feels *bruised when you brush your hair,* or your temples or the bridge of your nose may *hurt when you wear glasses.* Just one spot may be tender, or your whole scalp may *feel as if it's on fire.* Or your head may just be *sensitive.* Ironically, as much as your head, face or neck are *sore to the touch,* you may find relief by pressing on your temples or elsewhere around your head or neck, or by apply-

"My scalp is on fire!"

MARIA'S STORY

For two years, Maria experienced constant burning and itching of her scalp. It also felt tingly, tender and bruised. Sometimes it would turn red.

Maria had had headaches almost every day since she was a teenager—"sinus, migraines and maybe tension"—but these scalp sensations were something new. She had a number of blood tests and underwent two scalp biopsies, but no one could figure out what was going on—until a dermatologist sent her my way.

It was migraine. I advised Maria to eliminate Excedrin (Step 1 of the 1-2-3 Program) and also to avoid birth-control pills and dietary triggers (Step 2). In the beginning, she was very skeptical, though politely so.

She returned to see me after four months and told me she was "much, much better." And she was *much better,* across the board, with minimal scalp symptoms (when work became stressful) and mild eye pain only on the first day of her menstrual periods— all from taking a few simple steps. ◆

ing ice, thereby decreasing painful blood flow through swollen, inflamed vessels.

The discomfort produced by migraine can be one-sided and very focal—in just one spot inside or outside your head, face or neck, as in one eye or one ear. Or one whole side of your head, face or neck may hurt. But migraine pain is often diffuse and bilateral. Discomfort may be in the front, top or back of your head, or in your temples, forehead, sinuses, jaw or teeth.

Neck stiffness, aching, soreness, tightness and *tension* are common symptoms of migraine. You may experience what you call *knots* or *spasm* in your neck. It may feel as if *your head is too heavy* for your neck to support it. Your neck may *crack, creak, crunch, grind* or *pop.*

Discomfort often spreads into the trapezius muscles (located between your neck and shoulders) and into the shoulder blades in your upper back. The territory of migraine is broad, and the location of discomfort depends on the location of blood vessel swelling and inflammation.

Migraine can activate suddenly or gradually, with onsets ranging from explosive to insidious. The duration of discomfort generated by the mechanism of migraine ranges from split-second to continuous. You may experience *sudden, fleeting jolts* or *jabs, flashes of pain* or *stabbing ice-pick pains* here and there around your head. Such experiences often provoke concern about an aneurysm, brain tumor or impending stroke but are almost always migraine-related and benign (but for the unpleasantness of the pain itself).

On the other hand, migraine discomfort can last for weeks, months, years or even decades with no letup. The mechanism can be activated constantly on a long-term basis, as long as your trigger level exceeds your threshold. Migraine causes chronic daily headache—or neck ache, or sinus discomfort—in *many* people.

Chronic, persistent migraine usually has ups and downs: good days and bad days. When a person with chronic daily headache has a "good day," the level of trigger input is hovering just above the threshold. On a "bad day," it's soaring far above. For a chronic headache sufferer, a good day means that blood vessels are only mildly swollen and inflamed; a bad day means that the blood vessel disturbances—and consequent pain—are severe.

In short, migraine causes any kind of discomfort imaginable, anywhere in or around your head, face or neck. The headaches that are conventionally recognized as "migraines" are but a thin slice from the broad spectrum of headaches generated by the mechanism of migraine.

The Spectrum of Non-Headache Migraine

THE BROAD SPECTRUM of migraine headaches is echoed by the wide range of autonomic disturbances (*nausea, vomiting, constipation, diarrhea, flushing or pallor of the skin, sweating, chills* and *fever*) and the symptoms of inflamed meninges (photophobia, phonophobia and neck stiffness) that can occur to varying degrees and in different combinations . . . and with or without substantial head, face or neck discomfort. People sometimes mistakenly assume that headache pain itself produces nausea (and vomiting), but the truth is that migraine gives rise to both headaches and nausea independently. Some headache sufferers welcome the onset of vomiting, which for them heralds the end of a migraine episode. "Abdominal migraine" describes abdominal pain thought to arise from migraine, but in my view this is not very common.

Neurological symptoms of migraine, including visual disturbances, dizziness and many more, form a broad spectrum as well. As with all other aspects of migraine, the neurological symptoms vary extensively in degree and duration. Minutes-long is typical, but they may last split seconds, hours or longer—or even be constant for months or years. Often they commingle, or spread from one to another, as when flashing lights first appear, then give way to numbness of the face and tongue, or dizziness, or difficulty in speaking. There may or may not be accompanying head, face or neck discomfort, or autonomic dysfunction or meningeal symptoms, before, during or after the experience of neurological symptoms.

Neurological symptoms of migraine are far more common than is recognized, partly because they often occur in isolation, apart from headaches. While it is generally true that neurological symptoms are more likely when the migraine mechanism is highly activated, thereby also generating relatively severe headache and other symptoms, this rule is often broken. We can divide neurological symptoms of migraine into categories: visual, vestibular, auditory, somatosensory, olfactory, motor, cognitive, psychic and emotional arousal, seizure and stroke. Let's take a tour of this fascinating world of often peculiar and puzzling—yet surprisingly common—migraine experiences.

Visual Symptoms

CLASSIC VISUAL SYMPTOMS of migraine are unmistakable. If you have a *zigzag arc of flashing lights* gradually spreading across your field of vision and disappearing after 15 or 20 minutes, that's a textbook migraine "aura." But most visual symptoms of migraine are less dramatic. Vision may simply be *blurred, confused, difficult to focus, shaky* or *distorted* in a nonspecific way that is difficult to describe.

You may see *spots, dots, specks, flashing lights, sparkles, zigzags, lightning, squiggles, geometric shapes, jagged lines, chicken wire, rings, strings, shimmering, spiraling, halos, heat waves, ripples, clouds, cobwebs, bugs, amoebas, tadpoles, fish scales, TV static, holes, Picasso faces, ghosts* or *double images,* or you may have *tunnel vision.* These symptoms, especially when pain is absent, are referred to by some as ocular, ophthalmic, optical or retinal migraine.

Migraine is all the more likely the cause of visual symptoms when the symptoms are *bright, lively, colorful, scintillating* and *fleeting.* Symptoms often slowly expand outward or move around the field of vision. The site of blood vessel constriction associated with visual disturbances can be either the retina (the back of the eye, where light is registered), the occipital lobes of the brain (where vision is produced) or, with double vision, the brain stem (where eye movements are coordinated).

Photophobia, or sensitivity to bright light, arises from inflammation of meningeal blood vessels. Visual stimuli such as sunlight glare, fluorescent or flickering lights and ceiling fans may trigger migraine. With active migraine, some people find they can't tolerate supermarket aisles or malls, watching television or reading. Sometimes migraine causes the pupil of one eye to become larger or smaller, usually on the side of greater pain, and there may be drooping of the eyelid.

Vestibular Symptoms

NORMALLY, YOUR VESTIBULAR SYSTEM controls your balance by means of the fluid-filled semicircular canals in the inner ear. These peripheral sensors are connected by nerves to certain pathways and centers in the brain stem and elsewhere in the brain, and when vestibular function is disturbed by migraine, it may be felt as *unsteadiness, loss of equilibrium ("like just getting off a boat"), being off-balance, veering, swaying, falling, rocking, vertigo (a spinning sensation)*—or just vague, nonspecific *dizziness, lightheadedness* or *wooziness.*

Symptoms of migraine, especially these vestibular symptoms, are sometimes trigger-specific. Just as sunlight glare or a flashbulb going off in your face may specifically provoke a classic visual aura of flashing lights, so may the vestibular stimulation of moving your head rapidly or into a certain position cause vestibular symptoms of migraine. It has long been recognized that car sickness and other motion-induced ills are commonly related to migraine and reflect the heightened vestibular sensitivity of certain individuals, courtesy of their relatively low migraine thresholds.

As with all other neurological symptoms of migraine, vestibular symptoms can be transient or persistent and can occur with or without headache or other accompanying discomfort. The site of migraine-related blood vessel constriction causing dizziness can be either in the inner ear or in the vestibular pathways and centers of the brain. The

---

"My whole world seems out of kilter"

≈≈≈

ALICE'S STORY

S ometimes Alice saw "waves" off to the left—a warning that a severe headache was soon to follow. But for a month before coming to me, she'd had a "ghostlike" effect in her vision that made it seem as if what she saw with her left eye was "a frame behind" what she saw with her right eye.

Alice's headaches had worsened, too, with stabbing pain that began in her left eye, then spread to her right eye and around her head. She'd also had frequent feelings of being off-balance and two episodes of "the room spinning around" lasting 15 minutes.

These new symptoms occurred in a setting of stress following two deaths in the family, problems at work and a move into a new house—more or less simultaneously. All of what Alice felt was migraine, and it all responded well to a combination of dietary modification and a change in the medication she was taking for depression. We substituted the migraine-preventive antidepressant nortriptyline for Prozac, which in some people can stimulate migraine.

I've followed Alice for three years now, and not only has she continued to do well—with just mild headaches once in a while, and no dizziness—but she's also been able to eliminate her antidepressant medication without recurrence of migraine or depression. ◆

term "basilar migraine" is applied to intense episodes of migraine involving profound vertigo, imbalance, loss of consciousness and other symptoms arising from constriction of the basilar artery, which supplies the brain stem.

Auditory Symptoms

MIGRAINE CAN AFFECT the inner ear so as to produce auditory symptoms, including *tinnitus* (*ringing, buzzing* or some other *noise in the ear*) and *muffled hearing.* Even sudden hearing loss can occur. Again, these auditory symptoms, as with all neurological symptoms of migraine, can be momentary or prolonged, and may occur alone or in concert with headache and other symptoms. Phonophobia, or sensitivity to loud noise, is another auditory symptom of migraine.

Somatosensory Symptoms

SOMATOSENSORY SYMPTOMS of migraine include *numbness, tingling, pins and needles* and *falling-asleep feelings* on one or both sides of the head, face, neck or body. Facial symptoms are often described as feeling as if you've received an injection of Novocain at the dentist's office and it's wearing off. These symptoms reflect activation of the trigeminal nerve (usually on one side, but sometimes both), which not only plays a role in the mechanism of migraine but also supplies sensation to the face. Often the lips and tongue are affected. Similar feelings including *tingling, burning, coldness, pins and needles, itching, vibrations* or *water trickling* on one side of the back of the head represent activation of the occipital nerve, a branch of the cervical nerves through which migraine is expressed.

The somatosensory symptoms of migraine that involve the body may be on one side or both and often migrate within minutes from one location to another. This gradual spread of symptoms reflects a wave of blood vessel constriction traveling through the parietal lobes of the brain, where we experience sensation. Somatosensory symptoms generated in this way involve mainly the hands, less so the feet, and may also involve the arms, legs and face. People usually experience these symptoms as some type of numbness or tingling, but aching or other forms of discomfort in the limbs are sometimes felt.

Olfactory Symptoms

OSMOPHOBIA, OR SENSITIVITY to strong odors, occurs with migraine and is often associated with photophobia and phonophobia. Certain odors may also serve as migraine triggers, including perfumes, tobacco smoke, scented candles or incense, automobile "air fresheners" and cleaning products. (Some of my patients complain of "*Vogue* headaches" from contact with scratch-and-sniff perfume ads or can't tolerate the heavy aromas in certain stores.) Disturbance of olfactory (smell) sensation in migraine, most often *smelling a peculiar odor that isn't really there*, is less common and is caused by blood vessel constriction in the temporal lobes of the brain, which govern smell sensation.

Motor Symptoms

MOTOR SYMPTOMS OF MIGRAINE are usually subtle, such as *heaviness* or *clumsiness* of one hand and arm, but can include dramatic *weakness* mimicking a stroke. "Hemiplegic" and "complicated" migraine are terms applied to these stroke-like episodes, which stem from blood vessel constriction affecting the frontal lobes of the brain.

Cognitive Symptoms

COGNITIVE SYMPTOMS OF MIGRAINE range from common and non-specific—intermittent *trouble concentrating, spaciness, forgetfulness, difficulty finding words, not being able to think right*—to unusual and profound. For many people, migraine-related difficulty in concentrating is even more functionally disabling than headache, especially on the job.

"I couldn't breathe"

≋

SAUL'S STORY

Saul had experienced "scintillating rainbow vision" on a few occasions, triggered by combinations of heavy travel, stress, red wine, chocolate, processed meats and an "herbal decongestant" he sometimes took for "sinus" (episodes of pressure in his forehead, along with feeling off-balance and lightheaded). He figured that the visual symptoms were migraine, but he didn't get it that the so-called sinus stuff was, too.

What came next was a real surprise. Saul awoke in the middle of the night "with a jump" and felt "something terribly wrong." He was hot and sweaty. His hands tingled, his heart raced and he couldn't get enough air. In the midst of this, "rainbow vision" appeared; afterwards, his head hurt. Over the next few weeks, he had several similar but milder spells, and in between he felt dizzy and headachy all the time.

After all this, and before I met him, Saul had an extensive workup that led to a (mis)diagnosis of seizures. The antiseizure medication he took caused Stevens-Johnson syndrome, a potentially fatal allergic reaction in which his skin peeled off. Fortunately, he recovered . . . sort of. Saul would be the first to admit that he was kind of a mess when he first came to me with constant dizziness and headaches and a dreadful fear of another spell.

He isn't a mess anymore. For two years now, he's done, in his own words, very well. How? By recognizing that his problems were an interplay of migraine, panic attacks and anxiety, and by following the migraine-preventive diet. No more attacks, and the only times he's had headaches, including one "whopper" preceded by seeing what looked like "a bunch of tadpoles swimming in a petri dish" (Saul's a biology teacher), were when he pushed his luck too far in cutting corners on the diet. As he's gained control of migraine, he's also overcome his panic attacks and anxiety . . . drug-free. ◆

The most profound example of migraine-based cognitive impairment is transient global amnesia (TGA), during which an individual *loses memory for hours*. In an episode of TGA, you know who you are and you're able to perform most functions, but you can't remember the answer to a question asked moments earlier and afterwards recall nothing of the episode. Memory dysfunction from migraine relates to blood vessel constriction in the temporal lobes of the brain.

Psychic and Emotional Symptoms

STRANGE FEELINGS MAY PRECEDE, accompany or follow other, more overt symptoms of migraine. These feelings, which are often difficult to describe, may be ones of *dissociation* or *disconnection, otherworldly experiences, altered self-perceptions, vague premonitions* or *mood changes*— especially *depression*. Depression and migraine often cycle hand in hand, as if arising from a common origin in the brain. (Crying, not necessarily due to depression, can be a potent migraine trigger.)

Similarly interrelated are migraine and panic attacks. Panic attacks are sudden, overwhelming episodes of intense physical symptoms— *palpitations, difficult breathing, chest pressure, shaking, sweating, weakness, dizziness, numbness and tingling,* and others—accompanied by *fright*. The effects are like a powerful surge of adrenaline, the "fight or flight" hormone, and during a panic attack you may feel fearfully out of control.

Migraine can provoke panic attacks. Panic attacks can provoke migraine. Or the two may occur in concert, suggesting a shared source. Sometimes dizziness, tingling and other symptoms of migraine and panic attacks overlap, and it can be difficult to distinguish them.

Arousal Disturbances

DISTURBANCES OF AROUSAL with migraine vary widely from *sleepiness* or *lethargy,* often as a prelude to headache and other symptoms, all the way to sudden *loss of consciousness. Fatigue* is a major feature of

migraine, as is *yawning*. Brief, nonspecific loss of consciousness—
fainting—in otherwise healthy persons probably results from migraine
far more often than is recognized. When migraine causes fainting, the
activating system in the brain stem that regulates the brain's wakefulness malfunctions as a result of transient constriction of the blood vessels that supply it.

Seizures

THE BRAIN FUNCTIONS by means of highly controlled electrical activity.
During a seizure, the brain's electrical activity goes haywire; in other
words, a short circuit occurs. Seizures can happen for many reasons,
infrequently including migraine.

Any type of seizure may occur due to migraine, ranging from subtle episodes of *confusion* to dramatic *loss of consciousness* accompanied
by *stiffening and jerking of the limbs*. Seizures occur in migraine when
blood vessel constriction reduces flow to a part of the brain, and in
so doing, inhibits that part of the brain from maintaining its orderly
electrical activity.

Stroke

STROKE, LIKE SEIZURE, is an uncommon manifestation of migraine.
Instead of neurological deficits being transient, as is usually the case
with migraine, deficits from stroke are persistent, although over time
they may improve or resolve. Migraine-related blood vessel constriction, if sufficiently severe and prolonged, can lead beyond the point of
temporary dysfunction to actual death of brain tissue. Statistically, the
likelihood of stroke from migraine is remote.

Some people with migraine have persistent neurological symptoms lasting for days, weeks or longer, yet not because they've had a
stroke. That such episodes are not strokes is evident because the symptoms abruptly resolve when the migraine mechanism is turned off.

Moreover, even while symptoms are present, there is usually no damage to the brain detectable by sensitive studies including magnetic resonance imaging (MRI).

The Variety and Variability of Migraine

NOT ONLY WIDE VARIETY but also variability characterizes the symptoms of migraine. That is, your symptoms of migraine usually change over the course of your life.

You may be prone to episodic severe headaches that you recognize as migraine-related . . . and also to one or more kinds of mild-to-moderate, nonspecific headache that you regard as "tension" or "sinus" headache. You may also have neck stiffness that you think is arthritis or some other, altogether different issue. On top of this, you may have bouts of dizziness or fleeting visual disturbances, not necessarily associated with headache, that you don't even relate to your headache problem. Yet all these symptoms may stem from migraine as it becomes activated to varying degrees and expresses itself in multiple ways at different times.

Migraine can become problematic at any time of life, from early childhood through old age. Onset of symptoms is more common earlier than later, often beginning in the teenage years or early adulthood and, in women, most notably around menarche (the start of menstruation) or at other hormonal milestones (pregnancy, menopause). But migraine can also present in toddlers with attacks of vomiting and falling down. (Very young children may be unable to communicate their suffering and instead manifest migraine as irritability, fatigue, yawning, withdrawal, crying or just appearing pale and ill.) Elderly people also can experience chronic daily headaches, dizziness or visual disturbances for the first time after decades of only occasional, "normal" headaches.

As you go through life, migraine's manifestations are *likely to change*. In the past, right now or in the future, different kinds of dis-

Kids and Migraine

Comparing kids with adults, it's even *more* likely that children's headaches will be misdiagnosed as "psychosomatic" and blamed on school phobia, overachievement, parents' marital problems or a multitude of other factors. (Of course, these factors can serve as triggers for *migraine*, but not by causing "psychosomatic" head pain without a physical basis.) Likewise, childhood headaches are often incorrectly attributed to a "sinus" condition or to "eyestrain."

Teenagers with headaches need to resist the wayward pull of peers and their own biological makeup. Since a natural teenage tendency—to fall asleep late and wake up late—is reinforced by social pressures and reaches full bloom on the weekends, come Monday morning the child will be sleep-deprived and schedule-disordered. This may be why your child complains of headaches at school, *not* because it's an excuse to get out of class. The solution is to get enough sleep (8 to 10 hours is about right for a teenager) and to do so consistently, school night or not.

Discourage absences from school on account of headaches. You don't want your child to get into the bad habit of using headaches to shirk responsibility. You *do* want your child to achieve headache control, and that starts with staying in—not retreating from—the real world. Similarly, children should stay physically active while developing the means to prevent headaches, including those that exercise otherwise might tend to trigger. The point is to strive to maintain the normal childhood functions and activities while taking the right steps to gain control of headaches.

Many of the triggers listed in Chapter Four are staples of our children's diets, but self-discipline and the rewards of doing without provide a valuable life lesson that lasts into adulthood. Needless to say, it's also desirable to avoid having to add preventive medication for a child, but if this step is necessary, the dosage may need to be scaled down according to body size. ◆

comfort might afflict your head, face and neck. Over time, you may experience varying degrees of autonomic dysfunction, or neurological
symptoms that come and go—all arising from migraine and reflecting
its fluctuating nature. When overall migraine activity rises or falls, or
the pattern of migraine symptoms shifts, there must be one or more
reasons, but they may or may not be identifiable. In fact, often no reason is identifiable, probably because we're not smart enough to recognize it . . . or maybe because migraine sometimes has a mind of its own.

Changes in your overall migraine activity reflect changes in the
relationship between your threshold for activation and your trigger
load. Rises in overall migraine activity represent either a lower threshold
(genetically preprogrammed to occur at a certain time of your life or
brought on by a life event such as head trauma), increased trigger input
(which may or may not be recognizable), or both. Less easily explained
are shifts in the *nature* of migraine symptoms—for example, the new
appearance of flashing lights or dizziness—but the general trend toward
decreased headaches yet increased neurological symptoms of migraine
in the elderly points to age-related influences.

Throughout life, intermittent rises in overall migraine activity
and shifts in the pattern of migraine symptoms are the rule, not the
exception, but these changes are likely to worry you. When headaches
worsen, or you feel a new type of pain in a different part of your head,
you may imagine that a brain tumor is growing. An unprecedented
occurrence of brief, sharp pains in your head may make you think
you have an aneurysm that is about to burst. The development of
unfamiliar neurological symptoms such as flashing lights, dizziness, or
numbness and tingling of your face may provoke fear of stroke or
multiple sclerosis.

It's a good idea to check with your doctor if you're concerned
about increased or new symptoms. A serious problem *is* a possibility.
But most often these symptoms in an otherwise healthy person are

points on the broad spectrum of migraine—a spectrum that we all journey along in different ways and to varying degrees as we go through life.

Here's an all-too-familiar story. For whatever reason, recognizable or not, you have a rise or a change in migraine activity. But because you and your doctor don't realize that's what it is, your symptoms not only go untreated (or are mistreated), they worsen as your frustration, aggravation, confusion and anxiety grow, adding to your trigger burden. Understand migraine and deal with it properly, and this won't happen to you.

Before We Move On . . .

THIS IS A GOOD TIME TO PAUSE and consider where we are. I hope you've gotten the message so far: the world of migraine isn't flat; it's round— *big* and round—and we all live in it. Now, maybe you're not terribly bothered by headaches or any of the other symptoms that you now know stem from migraine. If that's true, then maybe it's not worth your while to do what you can do to control migraine, using the 1-2-3 Program outlined in the next three chapters.

But hold on. Could you be underestimating the scope of migraine in your life? Think of what you just learned from this chapter, and take stock of your own experience. Add up not only your headaches (of varying degrees) but also the pressure, fullness and heaviness in your head, plus your neck stiffness (which you figure is arthritis), your sinus congestion (which you chalk up to allergies), your dizziness and all the rest. These "low-grade" symptoms of migraine—which you thought you were stuck with, because whatever approaches you've tried haven't been very effective—are often *very chronic* and *nagging* and not really so low-grade after all.

Many people suffer from these kinds of symptoms with such regularity that they see them as facts of life, their burden to bear, a "necessary evil." Are you one of them? In order to cope, do you block out your awareness of these symptoms, even as they constantly lurk in the wings, ever ready to strike more forcefully, until finally they penetrate the radar screen of your consciousness when they get so bad that you simply can't ignore them any longer? The effort expended in trying to live with these chronic background symptoms is exhausting. No wonder so many people with active migraine problems—most of whom don't even recognize them as such—feel so tired all the time.

Although migraine is natural, it is *not* necessary. In fact, it's a treatment opportunity. You don't need to suffer from it, in any of its forms: episodic incapacitating headaches, chronic daily headache, neck stiffness, sinus congestion, dizziness or whatever. *You can control migraine*, as explained in the next three chapters, *but* your motivation to do the right things depends on the thoroughness of your personal inventory of migraine symptoms and their total impact on you (and those around you) and your life. Think about this carefully, feel the full measure of your personal migraine experience and you'll be better prepared to move on to Step 1.

One more thing: I suspect you might not like hearing some of what I have to say about the steps you must take to control your headaches. Especially the first step. Let's see if we can agree on something: if your headaches are a problem, whatever you're doing about them isn't working well. In fact, it may be making things worse. That means you need to do things differently. Right? Keep that in mind as you read on and take Step 1.

"Some days, I couldn't even get out of bed"

≈≈≈

TED'S STORY

Ted was preoccupied with "industrial-strength migraines" that sent him to bed two or three days each month. Finally he admitted that even on a "good day" he was "aware of something" in his head and that on most days he was embattled on two fronts: "sinus pressure" in his forehead and "tension" in his neck. It was when one of these forces surged that he became stricken and had to take to his bed.

As Ted initially saw it, that was the problem: the two or three days a month he couldn't function. As I saw it, the problem was vastly greater: encompassing every day, with relentless migraine activity—of varying degrees—that was diminishing his entire existence.

Ted just wanted one of the new quick fixes he'd heard so much about, maybe a triptan like Imitrex, to take on his bedridden days . . . on top of the Sinutabs and Anacin he was taking for his everyday discomfort. It wasn't easy, but I convinced him that rather than up his quick-fix dependence, it was worth his while to do certain things he didn't want to do—for starters, to eliminate all rebound-causing quick fixes (Step 1) and follow the migraine diet (Step 2)—in order to control the full spectrum of his migraine problem.

Ted took these steps and never looked back. His one regret was that he hadn't taken them sooner. Only after he had controlled all his headaches could he see clearly what I had seen from the beginning—that over the years he had become so accustomed to headaches that he had blocked out the vast majority and acknowledged only those that overwhelmed him. If you make that same mistake, you may not make the right decision—and take the right steps—to truly control your headaches. All of them. ◆

THE 1-2-3 PROGRAM

CHAPTER THREE

Step 1: Avoiding the "Quick Fix"

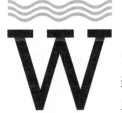

When you have a headache, you just want to get rid of it. If you're like most people, you rely on painkillers. If you use painkillers only infrequently, and they work, that's fine. But by taking certain quick fixes too frequently, you make your headache problem *worse* and more difficult to control. Avoidance of this complication, known as rebound, is what Step 1 is all about. But first let's look at how painkillers can be used appropriately, so that they don't make your headache problem even worse.

Acute Treatment of Migraine

Treating headaches with painkillers is appropriate only if the need arises infrequently, and only if the treatment is safe and effective. This means taking a safe and effective medication *at most* two days per month for severe headaches and *at most* two days per week for mild-

Acute Treatment of Mild-to-Moderate Headache

ACETAMINOPHEN (*without caffeine*)	up to 1,000 mg	every 4 hours
ASPIRIN (*without caffeine*)	up to 1,000 mg	every 4 hours
IBUPROFEN	200 to 800 mg	every 4 to 6 hours
NAPROXEN SODIUM	220 to 660 mg	every 6 to 8 hours

Table 1

to-moderate headaches. If your headaches are more frequent, or if your painkillers are adding to your problem (by causing rebound) or don't work well, you should concentrate on *preventing* your headaches rather than allowing yourself to be victimized and dependent on being rescued.

Acute treatment of mild-to-moderate headaches is simple—and should be kept that way (see Table 1, above). (With these and all other recommended medications, it's up to you and your doctor to weigh the potential benefits and risks to you.) The options listed are all available over the counter. Dealing with your headaches by taking one of these medications up to two days per week—*maximum*—is reasonable *if* it works. The earlier you take these drugs, and the higher the dosage, the better they work. It makes sense: these medications are anti-inflammatories that block activation of prostaglandins, chemicals that generate inflammation early in the course of migraine.

The medications in Table 1 are usually safe, but not 100 percent so. Acetaminophen can cause liver damage, especially with chronic, high-dose exposure. And with aspirin, ibuprofen and naproxen you run the risk of stomach irritation (or even bleeding) or kidney problems (particularly if you're predisposed by an underlying condition such as high blood pressure or diabetes). On the plus side, these med-

ications do not cause rebound, as do other quick-fix headache remedies. If your stomach's an issue, you might tolerate better one of the
newer, more selective anti-inflammatories available by prescription:
celecoxib (Celebrex) or rofecoxib (Vioxx). Other members of the large
family of anti-inflammatory drugs, available both over the counter and
by prescription, can be used interchangeably instead of ibuprofen or
naproxen but offer no substantial advantage and usually cost more.

When headaches occur, it can be helpful to eat something, to try
to relax, lie down in a dark, quiet room or go to sleep, to apply ice, heat
or gentle pressure, to be massaged, to do neck stretches or to exercise.
If you find any of these measures helpful, do whatever works for you as
soon as possible after a headache starts.

For *infrequent* severe headaches, triptans are the best acute treatment (see Table 2, page 40), but these drugs must be used no more than
two days per month or they'll lead to rebound. Triptans are "designer
drugs," in this case specifically designed to stimulate certain receptors
for the neurotransmitter serotonin. Remember that in the course of
migraine activation, nerve fibers release neuropeptides around blood
vessels, causing the vessels to become swollen and inflamed. When serotonin receptors located near the nerve terminals are bound by a properly fitting molecule, like a key in a lock, the release of neuropeptides is
blocked and therefore so is the blood vessel swelling and inflammation
that otherwise would result. Triptans are such molecules, designed to bind
to these serotonin receptors. Triptans also may work by binding to serotonin receptors in the brain stem and elsewhere, thereby interrupting the
mechanism of migraine at multiple sites.

All triptans come as tablets that act fairly similarly, with relatively
minor differences in effectiveness and side effects. Sumatriptan is also
available in self-injectable and nasal spray forms that are faster acting
than tablets. For some people, only the injectable form works. Approxi-
mately three-quarters of those who use a triptan obtain relief of headache,

Acute Treatment of Severe Headache

TRIPTANS		
SUMATRIPTAN (IMITREX)	25, 50 or 100 mg tablet	The original
SUMATRIPTAN	5 or 20 mg nasal spray	Faster than tablets
SUMATRIPTAN	6 mg self-injection	Fastest of all
NARATRIPTAN (AMERGE)	1 or 2.5 mg tablet	Relatively well tolerated
RIZATRIPTAN (MAXALT)	5 or 10 mg tablet (MLT form dissolves on tongue)	May be the best overall
ZOLMITRIPTAN (ZOMIG)	2.5 or 5 mg tablet	Similar to sumatriptan
ALMOTRIPTAN (AXERT)	6.25 or 12.5 mg tablet	The newest
OPIOIDS		
CODEINE	30 to 60 mg orally	
OXYCODONE	5 to 10 mg orally	

WARNING: Used more than two days per month, triptans and opioids can cause rebound. See text for details.

Table 2

nausea and photophobia (within an hour or so, if taken orally). Failure to respond to a triptan does *not* argue against the diagnosis of migraine.

Sometimes more than one dose of a triptan is required if headache recurs in a prolonged migraine episode. Triptans in tablet form are usually well tolerated, but sumatriptan injections and nasal spray are more likely to cause nuisance side effects including numbness, tingling, dizziness, flushing, and tightness of the throat or chest. (On the other hand, sumatriptan injections and nasal spray work faster and also may be preferable to triptan tablets when vomiting occurs along with headache.) All triptans carry a small risk of more serious complications, as discussed in the next section.

Treatment of Nausea and Vomiting

PROCHLORPERAZINE (COMPAZINE)	5 to 10 mg up to 3 or 4 times daily 25 mg up to twice daily	orally or intramuscularly rectally
PROMETHAZINE (PHENERGAN)	12.5 to 25 mg up to every 4 hours	intramuscularly, orally or rectally
TRIMETHOBENZAMIDE (TIGAN)	250 mg up to 3 or 4 times daily 200 mg up to 3 or 4 times daily	orally rectally
METOCLOPRAMIDE (REGLAN)	10 to 20 mg up to 4 times daily	intramuscularly or orally

Table 3

For patients with infrequent severe headaches who are at risk for complications of triptans or don't respond well to them, an opioid is the best alternative but also must be limited to no more than two days per month in order to avoid rebound. Used regularly, opioids (also known as narcotics) can lead to physical dependence and in some cases addiction, so that craving for the drug goes beyond its pain-relieving benefit.

Nausea and vomiting, whether associated with migraine or from other causes, can be relieved by drugs that block the action of the neurotransmitter dopamine (see Table 3, above). In the face of nausea and vomiting, these drugs are best administered by rectal suppository or injection. Especially when injected, dopamine antagonists may relieve not only nausea and vomiting but also headache. This means that in relieving headache these drugs are directly inhibiting part of the mechanism of migraine, indicating that dopamine, which they block, must be another neurotransmitter involved in the mechanism. Since dopamine antagonists don't cause rebound, they can be used safely (in that sense) for symptom relief, but of course they, too, have potential side effects, such as involuntary muscle contraction.

So much for the relatively good news about acute treatment of migraine. Now the bad news. The line between limited, *appropriate use* of acute treatment and *abuse* is a very fine one, which too many headache sufferers cross at considerable peril.

The Quagmire of Quick Fixes

LET'S TALK ABOUT THE PROBLEMS with quick fixes that you already know. To begin with, this approach means you have to have a headache before you can do anything about it. And then, you never really know if the quick fix is going to work. Or maybe you forgot to bring it with you, or you just realized, too late, that you've run out. All this unreliability increases your sense of insecurity—of being out of control, rather than in control. Not only do you worry about when a headache might strike, but you also don't know if you'll be able to get rid of it.

Side effects of quick fixes are sometimes mere nuisances, but other times they can be as incapacitating as the severe headaches they're intended to relieve. Triptans can aggravate nausea and vomiting, and—particularly in the case of sumatriptan by injection—can even make a headache worse. Although opioids may provide temporary pain relief, they also often cause disabling sedation. Rarely, side effects of quick fixes may be serious or even life-threatening, as when people with coronary artery disease use triptans, which may precipitate heart attack by constricting already narrowed arteries supplying the heart.

In addition, when migraine-related blood vessel constriction in the brain produces profound neurological symptoms such as paralysis on one side of the body, the situation may be worsened by triptans or other quick fixes that *further* constrict blood vessels. Although triptans may succeed in temporarily reducing painful blood vessel swelling around your head, there is concern that these drugs may also be capable of converting temporary insult (transient neurological symptoms of migraine) into permanent injury: stroke.

Victimization and Dependence

So MUCH FOR THE STRAIGHTFORWARD downsides of quick fixes. More importantly, but insidiously, they powerfully reinforce victimization and dependence. By relying on a quick-fix approach, you allow yourself to be victimized by headaches—rather than doing what you can to prevent them. When a headache strikes and has you in its clutches, you, the victim, are dependent on your quick fix for temporary rescue. At the same time, you also become dependent on the doctor who prescribes your rescue remedy.

What starts off simply—you and your doctor opting for the easy way out, following the path of least resistance and relying on painkillers—often gets complicated. You and your doctor may become entangled in a sticky web of victimization, dependence, blame and guilt. Initially the doctor may benefit from his or her role as rescuer. (Let me tell you, I've played that role, and it's a heady experience. It can be gratifying, even heroic, to relieve someone's suffering—even if only short-term.) And at the start the doctor-rescuer feels in control of providing you with short-term, apparent (but illusory) "control" of your headaches. Meanwhile you, the rescued victim, are grateful to the provider of your relief.

This arrangement may be fine at first, but soon the situation sours. Your headaches worsen because of rebound, as I'll explain shortly, and you come to depend ever more heavily on quick fixes. Your requests for quick fixes become more frequent, more urgent and more desperate. You feel more out of control, more dependent and more victimized, not only by headaches but also by your doctor, who has become uncomfortable with the situation and therefore reluctant to provide enough quick fixes to satisfy you.

The doctor also begins to feel a loss of control, being no longer the rescuer but now the unwitting victim of you and your burgeoning demands for drugs. Implicitly or explicitly, the doctor blames you, and in turn you feel guilty. Sensing that the doctor is blaming you, and feeling guilty because of it, you in turn blame the doctor for your deteriorating situation. The doctor, who already feels guilty because of caving in to your pleas for more drugs, feels even more torn and more guilty. The two of you become partners in a desperate dance, spinning out of control.

Quick Fixes Are Quicksand

A MORE TREACHEROUS and even more crippling problem with quick fixes is that they undermine your determination to do what you can do to prevent migraine. Preventive treatment—the 1-2-3 Program—can control your headaches and other migraine symptoms. But, in the beginning, preventive treatment often feels effortful and unrewarding. Unlike a quick fix, it is not immediately gratifying; establishing effective preventive treatment takes time and effort, at least at first. Once headache control is achieved, the steps taken to accomplish it become second nature, but first you need to gain headache control before you can reap the rewards of positive feedback.

If you have not yet achieved headache control, and an effective, well-tolerated quick fix is available, it becomes less likely that you will ever achieve headache control. A quick fix is an easy way out. You have an escape route, a detour. But the quick fix leads you astray, into a pool of quicksand, where you become stuck and struggle just to keep your head above water—or you sink below.

The right path is the (initially) uphill climb of preventive treatment, and if you take it you'll be glad when you reach the top and can see clearly the better life that lies ahead. If you take the easy way out instead, you'll never make it that far. For example, will you be sufficiently motivated to carefully modify your diet if you have a handy quick fix to rescue you from a severe headache that you bring on by eating or drinking something you shouldn't have? Likewise, your willingness to eliminate the birth-control pills or diet pills that may be contributing to your headaches—but that you want to take for other

"But my doctor keeps giving me what I ask for"

SHIRLEY'S STORY

I only saw Shirley twice. Her initial headache story was all too familiar. As a teenager she'd gotten by with B.C. Headache Powder around her periods. It eventually stopped working, and in her twenties Shirley graduated to the narcotic Darvocet: first once in a while, then a few times a week, and finally every day . . . more and more each day.

Shortly before we met, Shirley's doctor had prescribed OxyContin—an even more potent narcotic—because Darvocet wasn't doing the trick anymore. I tried my best to explain to Shirley that she had to give up drugs of this sort in order to gain control over her headaches. She listened, and I thought she got it.

But when Shirley returned in follow-up, she'd gotten nowhere. The doctor who was prescribing OxyContin told me he shared my concerns that it was counterproductive for Shirley, but he was either unable or unwilling to resist her requests. And even though Shirley wanted to stop, she couldn't seem to find the strength . . . at least, not while her doctor made OxyContin available.

I tried once more to reorient Shirley, to get her on the right track with the 1-2-3 Program. I never saw her again. I'm pretty sure I know what happened: because she wouldn't let go of OxyContin, her headaches would never let go of her. ◆

Are You a Candidate for Quick Fixes?

The rebound-causing quick fixes in Table 4 (page 47) should not be used by someone with frequent severe headaches. The appropriate candidate for quick fixes is the person with *infrequent* severe headaches—at most two days per month. This frequency may reflect a natural migraine tendency, or it may be a reduction from baseline, achieved in response to preventive treatment. If you previously suffered frequent, severe headaches and have achieved reasonable headache control with preventive treatment but still have severe breakthrough headaches infrequently, you *may* now be a candidate for a quick fix. But be careful: these quick fixes put you on a slippery slope, and you can easily backslide out of control. ◆

reasons—is eroded by quick fixes that let you cope with your headaches short-term. Should daily preventive medication be necessary for you to achieve headache control, your tolerance of initial nuisance side effects may be undermined if a quick fix is available to get you by, even if only one day at a time.

Overcoming your dependence on quick fixes and controlling your headaches requires long-range perspective. You must recognize the full extent of your current (and former) suffering, multiply that as you look years ahead down the long, wrong, downhill path you're on, and find the motivation to get on the right path and gain control. You have to be able to see farther than your nose and not just ask, *What can I take the next time I get a headache?*

Rebound: The Real Culprit

INSIDIOUS AND CUMULATIVE, rebound is the single biggest problem with quick fixes and the greatest potential impediment to headache control. Here's how it works. You take a quick fix to relieve a headache. The quick fix helps temporarily. As the quick fix wears off, your headache tendency increases. You bask in the glow of short-term headache relief, but rebound is a dark cloud on the horizon. Thanks to rebound, your headaches keep going—and growing.

Quick Fixes That Cause Rebound

CAFFEINE-CONTAINING ANALGESICS	Excedrin, Anacin, Vanquish, B.C. Headache Powder, Fiorinal, Fioricet, Esgic Plus and others
BUTALBITAL COMPOUNDS	Fiorinal, Fioricet, Esgic Plus, Phrenilin and others
ISOMETHEPTENE COMPOUNDS	Midrin, Duradrin and others
DECONGESTANTS	Sudafed, Tylenol Sinus, Dristan, Afrin, Entex LA and *many* others—both over-the-counter and by prescription
ERGOTAMINES	Ergomar, Wigraine, Migranal and D.H.E. 45
TRIPTANS	Imitrex, Amerge, Zomig, Maxalt, Axert and others soon to follow
OPIOIDS AND RELATED DRUGS	Tylenol with codeine, Percocet, Darvocet, Stadol NS, OxyContin, Ultram and many others

Table 4

Rebound Takes You Prisoner

REBOUND DEVELOPS over weeks, months or years. It is usually not evident in the short run, from dose to dose of a quick fix. (When headache recurs as a quick fix wears off, it may simply represent a continuation of the original headache.) Instead, rebound *gradually* promotes increased headache frequency and severity. It is rarely recognized—at least to its full extent—by the person caught in its vicious cycle. Each headache leads to another quick fix, and each quick fix leads to the next headache, and so on.

As rebound develops, you might wake up with headaches earlier and earlier as a sign that overnight you're withdrawing (and rebounding) from your quick fix. Or, indicative of the way rebound not only heightens headache tendency but also fosters drug resistance, you might find yourself less responsive to a quick fix that used to work well for you.

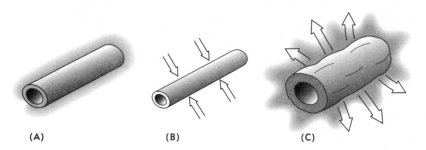

(A)   (B)   (C)

FIGURE 4: REBOUND VASODILATION. *Migraine causes blood vessels to swell (A). Certain drugs act on these blood vessels by constricting them (B), thus temporarily alleviating the painful swelling. When the drug wears off, the blood vessels react by swelling to an even greater degree than in the first place (C).*

How do quick fixes cause rebound? Most work by constricting the blood vessels around your head that become swollen due to migraine. You can imagine what happens when the formerly swollen blood vessels escape from the temporary, artificial constriction brought on by the drug. They swell *with a vengeance* in a process known as rebound vasodilation (see Figure 4, above).

Opioids (and related drugs that bind to opiate receptors) are quick fixes that don't constrict blood vessels but *do* cause rebound through a different mechanism. Opioid rebound involves changes in the receptors for these drugs. Normally when an opiate receptor is bound by a drug, the result is reduction of the noxious quality of pain . . . until the drug wears off. When opiate receptors are bound by opioids too frequently, the receptors become so accustomed to being bound that in a sense they can't stand being unbound, or naked. As a result, the absence of receptor binding (whenever the drug wears off) leads to *increased* pain, or rebound. It's as if the receptors are "crying out" for more drugs in order to satisfy their "desire" to be bound again. And in order to

"Each new drug was a lifesaver . . . until the roof caved in"

BERNADINE'S STORY

*I*n the beginning, Bernadine's headaches came only once or twice a month, and the Fiorinal she got from her mother—also a headache sufferer—worked great. The thing was, Bernadine's headaches kept coming more often and getting worse. Before she knew it, she was using Fiorinal just about every day. The doctor she'd found to prescribe it wasn't too happy about that, and neither was Bernadine—especially because the Fiorinal wasn't working so well anymore.

That's when Imitrex came along: a godsend, because it really worked. For a while. And then, wouldn't you know it, the Imitrex didn't work so well anymore, either. Plus, Bernadine's headaches were worse than ever.

No wonder. Bernadine was rebounding to beat the band. It wasn't easy for me to convince her that she had to get rid of Imitrex—and not substitute another rebound-causing drug in its place—but she was desperate and finally gave in.

In time, Bernadine came to feel she was living a new life, nearly free of headaches—just a "premonition" now and then— and completely free of drug dependence. Although initially she stuck with the migraine-preventive diet, eventually she drifted away from it. Yet she didn't suffer recurrent headaches, indicating that her once-active migraine tendency had subsided—perhaps long ago—and that rebound had been the main driving force behind her persistent severe headaches for many, many years. ◆

The Power to Please

Why do doctors inappropriately prescribe rebound-causing quick fixes? Three reasons stand out: (1) Many doctors are unaware of the rebound effect of quick fixes. (2) These drugs can be almost magical in their ability to quickly (though only temporarily) relieve suffering, and it's a powerful feeling to prescribe them. I know. *I* feel the power when I occasionally prescribe them (*appropriately*, I hope). (3) Quick fixes are an easy way out. Doctors don't like telling people what they don't want to hear—*Sorry, no more quick fixes*—and don't like unhappy customers storming out through their waiting rooms complaining loudly of mistreatment. Refilling quick-fix prescriptions again and again fulfills everyone's needs—for the short term. ◆

shut them up—and get rid of your rebound headache—you take another dose of the drug and become increasingly dependent and ever more headache-prone.

If quick fixes are used infrequently, no more than two days per month, the long-term consequences of rebound do not develop. The increased headache tendency that follows each exposure to a quick fix eventually subsides over days to weeks, and these increments don't add up and cause rebound—*if* enough time lapses between doses. When consumption of quick fixes rises to several times per month, too often the rate soon becomes once or twice per week, then several times per week, then more or less daily, as rebound takes you prisoner.

Rebound Cripples You

IT'S BAD ENOUGH that rebound increases headache frequency and severity. What's worse is that rebound blocks your ability to respond to preventive treatment. Preventive treatment—Steps 2 and 3 of the 1-2-3 Program—can put the brakes on your headaches. If rebound is driving your headaches forward, the brakes—preventive treatment—will fail. Your headache problem will continue to career downhill, and you won't be able to stop it. No matter what you do to try to prevent your next headache, rebound will guarantee it. As long as rebound is around, your headache problem is immortal.

Most of my new headache patients have been previously labeled as "failed" headache patients. Supposedly they have intractable headaches that are resistant to every treatment under the sun. According to these patients and their referring doctors, they have been everywhere and done everything to treat their headaches, all to no avail.

Almost without exception, these patients have never had a fair trial of *proper* preventive treatment. The guidelines for preventive treatment are spelled out in the next two chapters, but the first rule is this: *You need to eliminate rebound before you can respond to preventive treatment.* You can try preventive medications from now to eternity—maybe you feel as if you already have—but in the face of rebound preventive treatment won't work.

The stories most of my headache patients tell me are remarkably similar. In the beginning, there was a certain level of headache frequency and severity—not too bad—and the patient began using over-the-counter quick fixes. Plain acetaminophen, aspirin or ibuprofen weren't very effective, but Excedrin or a decongestant (for "sinus" headache) worked for a while. Eventually, as rebound developed, headache frequency and severity increased and response to these quick fixes waned.

Over the years, these patients had climbed a ladder of quick fixes including prescription drugs such as Fiorinal, Midrin, Tylenol with codeine, Percocet, Cafergot and Imitrex. Urgent visits to the doctor's office or trips to an emergency room for injections became part of an escalating pattern. Along the way, one or more doctors thought migraine might be part of the problem and prescribed preventive medications, none of which worked well and many of which were tolerated poorly. Looking back, there were lots of mistakes made with these preventive medication trials—incorrect drugs, inadequate (or excessive) dosages

Can Over-the-Counter Medications Cause Rebound?

Plain acetaminophen, aspirin and anti-inflammatory drugs such as ibuprofen and naproxen do not cause rebound. But caffeine-containing versions of them (such as Excedrin) do.

You might argue that the simple painkillers don't work and Excedrin Migraine does. Yes, the addition of caffeine to acetaminophen and aspirin (as in Excedrin and certain other over-the-counter pain-killers such as Anacin, Vanquish and B.C. Headache Powder) may help relieve headaches acutely, because caffeine constricts blood vessels. And, for the same reason, caffeine promotes rebound. If you have infrequent headaches and use a drug such as Excedrin infrequently—*no more than two days per month*—no problem. If you use it more frequently, you're asking for trouble.

Caffeine-containing painkillers aren't the only over-the-counter drugs that can cause rebound. Decongestants in "sinus" medications also constrict blood vessels, thereby acutely relieving symptoms of migraine (including not only headache but also sinus congestion) in the short run while leading to rebound in the long run.

You don't need a doctor's prescription in order to rebound. You can do it all by yourself, off the shelves of your friendly neighborhood pharmacy. ◆

and failure to reduce exposure to avoidable triggers—but above all it was rebound that doomed these trials to failure from the start.

At some point, both patient and doctor(s) gave up on further trials of preventive medication and resigned themselves to the notion that a quick-fix approach was the best they could do; otherwise the patient would be left to suffer with chronic headaches with no help at all. Thus the patient became certified as a "failed" headache patient and eventually arrived at my door. But it's not the patient who's a failure. Failure is the predictable result of quick-fix treatment and the rebound that it causes.

What's the Solution?

IDEALLY, REBOUND should be avoided in the first place by limiting the use of rebound-causing quick fixes (see Table 4, page 47) to two days per month. But once the problem has developed, the solution is simple: rebound must be eliminated, and this means eliminating the quick fixes that are causing it. You must stop taking rebound-causing quick fixes altogether in order to become responsive to preventive treatment. You must clear your system, which in its natural state—uncontaminated by rebound—*will* respond to preventive treatment. What you want in the long run is headache control, and this can be achieved only by giving up what you want in the short run: quick fixes.

I can hear you say, *You must not understand my suffering!* Let me reassure you, I do. I understand not only how much you suffer in the throes of a terrible headache, but also (and more so) how much you suffer overall, and will continue to suffer, living with an out-of-control problem. You can gain control only if you start by eliminating rebound. Then you can begin to leave your suffering behind.

In a *perfect* world, a chronic headache sufferer who is rebounding might be able to follow a preventive treatment program, eventually respond to it despite continued use of quick fixes as needed and then walk away from the quick fixes effortlessly and painlessly once headache control is achieved. But ours is not a perfect world. In *this* world, as long as you depend on quick fixes and therefore experience rebound, you will not respond to preventive treatment. You have to divorce yourself from quick fixes—that's Step 1—in order to achieve headache control by means of Steps 2 and 3.

What <u>Can</u> You Take for a Severe Headache?

If you get severe headaches more than infrequently, this is a bad question because it has only bad answers: quick fixes that will keep you trapped in rebound.

Any drug likely to satisfy you temporarily in the face of a severe headache will cause rebound. If in the process of trying to eliminate rebound you switch from one rebound-causing quick fix to another, you simply perpetuate rebound under a different name. The more effective a quick fix, the greater rebound it causes. Quick fixes are double-edged swords, and the higher-potency quick fixes are sharper in cutting both ways.

In place of the rebound-causing quick fixes, you can take plain acetaminophen or aspirin (without caffeine), or anti-inflammatories such as ibuprofen or naproxen (Table 1, page 38). These drugs are unlikely to satisfy you fully as you withdraw from quick fixes, but at least they don't cause rebound. (And once your headaches are under control but may be still occurring once in a while, these drugs are likely to work just fine.) You may also use medication to control nausea and vomiting (Table 3, page 41), and injectable versions of this type of medication are sometimes effective in relieving headache, too.

Instead of asking, *What can I take when I get a severe headache?* ask, *How can I prevent my headaches?* That's a *good* question with a *good* answer: the 1-2-3 Program. And see if you can't turn a negative into a positive: each time you have a headache and forgo quick fixes, let your suffering strengthen your resolve to do what you can do to *prevent* the next. ◆

I realize that the prospect of eliminating rebound by getting rid of quick fixes may feel scary and overwhelming. But you *must* do it, and you *can* do it. Be brave, be tough and have faith in yourself.

Look, if rebound is part of your headache problem, you have two options. The first, a *bad* choice, is to stay on your present downhill course until you reach bottom. As long as rebound persists, you will remain the captive of your headache problem. The other, *good* choice is to gain control of your headache problem, and the first step is to give up rebound-causing quick fixes. Admittedly, elimination of rebound may be difficult. First, you have to get rid of the crutches that you've been leaning on—and without which you may find it difficult to imagine being able to stand alone. But you *can* stand without your quick fixes. The truth is, *it's your crutches that are crippling you.* You can't walk on your own until you get rid of them.

The second reason that elimination of rebound may be difficult is that withdrawal can cause your headaches to increase for a few days or even up to a few weeks. Withdrawal headaches occur initially in about half my patients. In some cases, elimination of rebound is less troublesome or even trouble-free, but you must be psychologically and emotionally prepared for the possibility of a temporary, rough transition as you leave rebound behind and thereby open the door to headache control.

As difficult as it may be to get through this temporary transition, remember: *it's temporary.* Of my many patients who have toughed this out, I can't think of one who, after the fact, regretted it. Again, it's temporary, whereas the headache control you can gain is *permanent.*

The need to eliminate rebound may sound like bad news, but if you listen carefully to my message, it's *good* news. The message is: *You can control your headaches!* It starts with getting rid of your quick fixes. The short-term price you may pay as you cast your crippling crutches aside is well worth the long-term rewards of headache control. It'll be the best investment you'll ever make, and it's an investment in *yourself.*

You might want to say you can't do it right now—you're in the middle of something important, or you have something coming up. There will never be a good time to eliminate rebound. (When is there ever a good time to do something we should or must do, but don't want to?) But the time is now. It's the right thing to do, and each day you put it off lessens the likelihood that you will ever do it.

Cold Turkey vs. Tapering Off

TO ELIMINATE REBOUND, I recommend the "cold turkey" approach except in uncommon instances where abrupt withdrawal might be dangerous, as with daily dependence on high-dose narcotics or certain other drugs. Check with the doctor prescribing your quick fix(es) to make sure that stopping abruptly is safe.

True, tapering your reliance on quick fixes sounds easier than stopping abruptly and may dampen the increased headaches and other unpleasant symptoms that can accompany "cold turkey," but gradual withdrawal has a major flaw: It tends never to end. Despite your best intentions, you might easily find that your plan to cut back on your drug reliance instead sputters and stalls. You may never reduce your quick-fix consumption enough to escape from rebound, which guarantees your next headache, for which you take the next quick fix . . .

Picture yourself standing next to a large oak tree with a thick rubber belt looped around the tree trunk and around your waist. The tree represents quick fixes, and the rubber belt is your dependence on them. You want and *need* to eliminate your dependence on quick fixes, and you can do that by cutting the rubber belt and walking away. But instead you try walking away from the tree while still connected to it by the rubber belt. What happens? The tension of the belt steadily increases, making it harder and harder for you as you try to walk farther away, until finally the tension becomes so great that it snaps you back against the tree. You're right back where you started. Unless you make a clean break from quick fixes, the force they exert over you as you attempt to withdraw slowly tends to overcome you.

My new patients who are rebounding and who agree to tackle the problem nonetheless often try to bargain for reduced rather than zero

Hospitalization for Headaches?

Hospitalization to facilitate withdrawal from rebound or for acute headache relief is best avoided unless absolutely necessary (as *may* be the case with withdrawal from high-dose dependence on certain drugs). The problem of rebound stems from dependence on rescue therapy. Hospitalization is the *ultimate* rescue, and it sends the wrong message. It says you can't control yourself and your headache problem; you need other people to rescue you. The message should be that once you understand the problem of rebound, you can eliminate your quick fixes *yourself*.

Moreover, trials of preventive medications undertaken in the hospital are fatally flawed. Ongoing rebound from quick fixes (or withdrawal headaches from recent elimination of quick fixes) undermines your ability to respond to preventive medications. Time constraints on hospitalization demand that preventive medications be given "too much, too soon" and for too short a time. A preventive medication that fails under these circumstances may never be revisited, even though it may have worked well if used in the proper, outpatient setting. And even if headache control is achieved in a hospital, the factors responsible may not be transferable to the outside world. Hospital-dependent headache control is transitory, whereas headache control that *you* establish in the *real* world can last a lifetime.

A common justification given for hospitalization is "to break the headache cycle" with medication such as intravenous D.H.E. 45 (dihydroergotamine). This is all wrong. Experiencing chronic headaches does not preclude effective preventive treatment of them. The cycles that must be broken are those of victimization and dependence, blame and guilt—and the vicious cycle of rebound. Hospitalization for D.H.E. 45, another quick fix capable of causing rebound but masquerading as a unique rescue therapy, only reinforces these cycles. ◆

consumption of their quick fix: *Why can't I just take it twice a month, when I have my really bad headaches?* Three reasons. First, they'll probably find excuses to use it more than that, especially if they experience withdrawal headaches as they reduce their quick-fix consumption. Second, if they still have an easy way out of trouble, they'll be less likely to stick with preventive treatment—which may feel unrewarding and seem difficult at first. Third, even if they do comply with preventive treatment, they may not respond well if they don't escape far enough from rebound to be *able* to respond well.

If you're rebounding, I say: *Flush your quick fixes down the toilet, where they belong.* These drugs are *not* your best buddies; they're your *worst enemies.* By flushing them, you're declaring that you believe in yourself and your ability to gain control over your headaches and headache treatment. In a sense, although there will still be battles to fight, you'll have already won the war. On the other hand, by *not* throwing away your quick fixes, you're allowing your self-doubt to become a self-fulfilling prophecy—and you're perpetuating your headaches' control over *you* rather than achieving control over *them.*

As with so many things in life, long-term gain comes with short-term pain. When my patients return for their first follow-up, after having eliminated rebound and taken the necessary other steps to achieve headache control, they may mention—in passing—that it was rough for a few weeks in the beginning. But mainly they want to talk about how much better they are and how wonderful it feels to have control.

After the Dust Settles

ONCE YOU'VE ELIMINATED REBOUND and achieved stable, long-term headache control by means of preventive treatment, there is the *possibility* that a quick fix can eventually be reintroduced for severe breakthrough headaches that may still occur infrequently—but no more than two days per month. For some people this may be safe. But for others the reintroduction of quick fixes at *any* time may be as dangerous as a recovering alcoholic's having a drink to celebrate an anniversary of abstinence. You can decide for yourself down the road, after you've achieved headache control and can better judge how secure you are in it.

Elimination of rebound is potentially the hardest but also the most important step toward controlling your headaches. Taking Step 1 alone probably won't resolve your headache problem, but once you've accomplished this challenge, you'll be able to benefit from Step 2 and, if needed, Step 3. And if rebound is not already a part of your headache problem, consider yourself fortunate and *stay away from the trap*: don't use a rebound-causing quick fix more than two days per month.

CHAPTER FOUR

Step 2: Reducing Your Triggers

Now that you understand the mechanism that causes headaches and have learned the importance of avoiding quick fixes and their counterproductive rebound effect, you're ready to take control. By reducing your migraine trigger level, you can change your life. You may be amazed at how readily you can control your headaches (and other symptoms of migraine) simply by modifying your diet. For many longtime headache sufferers, the response is little short of miraculous.

The key is understanding how this approach works—and why you haven't figured it out for yourself. Telling you what to do isn't enough. Instead, as you read on, you'll come to know not only *what* you should do, but *why* you should do it. Now let's get to work . . .

Remember, when you experience headaches or other symptoms of migraine, it's because your trigger level has exceeded your threshold. The higher your trigger level climbs above your threshold, the more

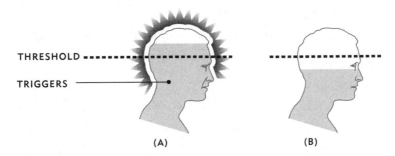

THRESHOLD

TRIGGERS

(A)   (B)

FIGURE 5: REDUCING YOUR TRIGGER LOAD. *When your trigger level rises above your threshold (A), you experience headaches or other symptoms of migraine. The good news is, you can lighten your trigger load and be symptom-free (B) by modifying your diet and avoiding certain medications.*

fully activated the mechanism and the more severe your symptoms. Controlling your headaches and other symptoms of migraine is simple: you just have to keep your trigger level below your threshold.

Step 2, reducing your trigger load, may be all it takes (see Figure 5, above). Reducing your trigger load is accomplished primarily by avoiding certain dietary items and medications. If this approach alone doesn't achieve satisfactory control of symptoms, you can take Step 3, the final step of preventive treatment: raising your threshold by using preventive medication, as explained in the next chapter.

How Triggers Add Up

THERE ARE MANY TRIGGERS for migraine, within and around us. And a number of these triggers are unavoidable—or at least difficult or undesirable to avoid (see Table 5, page 62). There's little you can do, for example, to avoid changes in barometric pressure, such as those that occur in an airplane cabin or when a storm approaches. If you're a

Unavoidable or Difficult-to-Avoid Migraine Triggers

BAROMETRIC PRESSURE & WEATHER CHANGES:
Approaching storms
Heat and humidity
Air travel
High altitude

HORMONAL FLUCTUATIONS:
Menstrual cycle
Pregnancy
Menopause

SENSORY STIMULI:
Perfumes
Tobacco smoke
Cleaning products
Bright light

PHYSICAL EXERTION:
Bending over
Aerobic exercise
Weight lifting
Coitus
Dehydration

SLEEP DEPRIVATION

STRESS

Table 5

woman, for much of your life you bear the ongoing burden of estrogen as a trigger, and to make matters worse you're naturally subject to hormonal fluctuations (especially falling estrogen levels) that tend to stimulate migraine around your menstrual periods and during menopause. While you personally can avoid wearing perfumes and using certain cleaning products—among the many odorants that commonly, powerfully and often suddenly trigger migraine—you may not be able to avoid exposure outside the privacy of your home.

And though you can make efforts to avoid triggers such as sleep deprivation, stress, depression or strenuous physical exertion, often these situations occur despite your best intentions or even on an intentional basis, as when you choose to work out or have sex and suffer a predictable headache as a consequence. But, for good reasons, you still want to work out and have sex. And you *can*, without suffering headaches, if you manage certain other triggers differently.

Unavoidable triggers are worth recognizing, if only because they stack up with more avoidable ones. For instance, several triggers inherent in air travel—long lines, security concerns, pesky flight delays (and cancellations!), luggage worries, barometric pressure changes in airplane cabins and sleep

Choosing Your Battles

It's true that you could help control your headaches by getting enough sleep, managing stress better and avoiding certain physical activities that provoke your headaches. It's also true that neither do I specifically counsel my first-time patients in these regards, at least not in the beginning, nor will I belabor these issues with you.

Why not? Because you have to choose your battles. If you try to fight too many at once, you won't win enough (if any) and you'll lose the war. Faced with a long laundry list of too many lifestyle changes and other steps to take, odds are you won't take any of them because you'll be confused and overwhelmed. You have to choose just a few battles: the ones most worth fighting.

Fact is, for many people who don't get enough sleep, and for most who are overly stressed, there isn't a great deal they can readily do about these problems. And while certain headache-provoking physical activities such as exercise or sex could be avoided, doing so would substantially reduce the overall quality of life, even if headaches were diminished as a result.

So let's focus on two battles in particular: (1) avoiding rebound, and (2) reducing your exposure to certain dietary and medication triggers. Why? Because you can win these battles, and by doing so you'll win the war to control your headaches. And even if your victory isn't perfect, you will nonetheless be in a much better position to begin dealing with some of these other issues, such as getting more sleep or managing stress, that would only help to further control your headaches.

Once you're in control, by means of the 1-2-3 Program, you'll be able to find your own way to a better life in more ways than just fewer headaches. You will see more clearly the right directions for you to take, and be able to take them, on your own. ◆

Weekend Headaches

Weekend headaches are one more example of the way that unavoidable *and* avoidable triggers stack up. Letdown from the stress of the workweek can be a trigger, and one that can't be avoided easily (unless you want to keep working all weekend, too). But weekend headaches also arise from oversleep on weekend mornings, excessive alcohol intake on Friday and Saturday nights, and caffeine withdrawal (from drinking less coffee on weekends than on weekdays). All of these triggers *can* be addressed. If you suffer from weekend headaches, you can help avoid them by getting up at the same time on Saturday and Sunday as on weekdays, not drinking too much alcohol and *eliminating caffeine altogether.* ◆

disturbances (especially with time zone changes) add together and predispose you to headaches. But *by themselves*, these unavoidable triggers may not reach above your threshold and give you a headache. If you avoid the many migraine-triggering foods and beverages found in airports and on airplanes—and by doing so avoid adding these items to your stack of unavoidable triggers—you can keep your total trigger level below your threshold and not get a headache. Similarly, hormonal fluctuations, especially with menstrual periods, are vulnerable situations that may necessitate reducing your exposure to additional, *avoidable* triggers in order to prevent headaches at those times.

Avoidable triggers are, for the most part, things that are swallowed: certain foods and beverages, and medications. (Perhaps surprisingly, tobacco and marijuana don't seem to be important triggers—at least, not for the smoker.) But you may be wondering why, if you've suffered from headaches all these years, you haven't been able to recognize for yourself that your diet is contributing to the problem. Or why, at best, you've recognized a few items and *still* suffer despite avoiding them.

It turns out that there are several good reasons for this.

Why Dietary Triggers Go Unrecognized

THE EXTENT TO WHICH FOODS and beverages contribute to headaches escapes most headache sufferers. (In contrast, we are strongly inclined to associate what we eat or drink with subsequent nausea and vomiting, even if an unrelated stomach virus is the actual culprit.) Sometimes individuals recognize that a few items, such as chocolate, red wine and Chinese restaurant food, occasionally (but typically not always) trigger headaches. These items are the tip of an iceberg. If certain dietary triggers have stood out in your experience, you might assume that all dietary triggers would be so obvious, but that's *not* the case.

One reason headache sufferers don't more fully appreciate dietary triggers is the potential delay of hours—*or up to a day or two*—from the time an item is consumed until its impact is felt. It's as though the migraine control center has a temporary "memory" for recent exposure to dietary triggers and can store their influence beyond their actual presence in your system. It's true that sometimes dietary triggers act quickly, within minutes, but often they don't, and this delay obscures their recognition.

Another reason dietary triggers go unrecognized is that even when you notice that *sometimes* an item is followed by headaches, you also notice that sometimes it's *not*, leading you to the mistaken conclusion that it must not be a factor, or at least not much of one. It's sort of logical to think that a trigger would cause a headache every time you ate or drank it, but that logic fails to take into consideration the fluctuating level of all your other triggers.

Imagine that one day your total trigger level is just below your threshold. You've been under a lot of stress, you didn't sleep well last night and there's a storm approaching. You're on the verge of migraine activation and its consequences, including headache, but you don't realize this since you don't have a meter that warns, *Hey, be*

Sex and Headaches

Sex-related headaches are fairly common, often occurring with orgasm. These headaches tend to be briefly excruciating, then linger at a lower level, and typically concerns arise that they may be due to an aneurysm or some structural problem in the brain. That's rarely the case; rather, it's migraine.

One treatment approach might be to advise against sex—or at least against orgasm. But this is a good example of a potentially avoidable trigger that is undesirable to avoid. What can be done instead? It's simple. You can avoid *other* triggers—ones that aren't so undesirable to avoid— in order to reduce your total trigger level.

Here's a letter from one of my patients, Ron, who wrote:

"For two months, every time I reached climax, I'd get a severe headache—a '10'— that felt like my heart beating in my head. I used to have what I figured were sinus headaches, but nothing like this. So I followed your advice and stopped caffeine completely. (So did my wife, by the way.) I didn't have caffeine withdrawal. And it's miraculous: no more headaches with sex! Or at all—not even sinus headaches!"

Sometimes you can avoid headaches provoked by specific exertion such as sexual activity (or weight lifting or jogging) by taking an anti-inflammatory medication such as ibuprofen or naproxen shortly beforehand. A relatively high dose (Table 1, page 38) may be required and can be repeated post-activity. ◆

careful! You're near the red zone! That day you indulge in chocolate. *Mmmm, it tastes good.* It's also a trigger, and that day it raises your total trigger level from just below threshold to well above (see Figure 6, page 67). Sooner or later you get a nasty headache, and especially if it's relatively soon, you may think, *Darn,* because you've heard that chocolate can trigger headaches and maybe it just did. But because

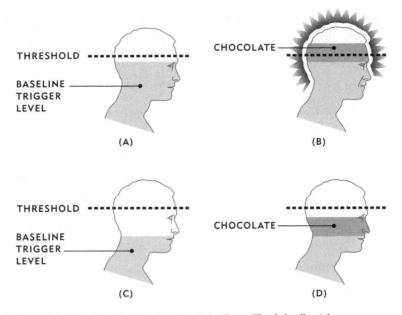

FIGURE 6: BAD DAYS vs. GOOD DAYS. *On a "bad day," with a near-threshold trigger level to start (A), a dietary trigger such as chocolate can raise the level to a point where migraine is activated (B). On a "good day," with a low trigger load to start (C), that same dietary trigger will fail to push the total level above your threshold (D) and you'll stay headache-free.*

---

you enjoy chocolate so much—and don't want to face the fact that you should avoid it in order to control your headaches—you give it another try a few days later. This time you don't get a headache! And you breathe a deep sigh of relief, not realizing that you've just been fooled.

The difference is that this time you had a lower level of other triggers beforehand. You were feeling less stress, you'd had a good night's sleep and the weather was better. But you don't realize that the reason you didn't get a headache that day is that you had plenty of margin for error. The addition of chocolate raised your trigger level, just like before, but this time there was lots of room below the threshold to start, so you didn't cross the line.

Instead of understanding that you were just lucky this time, you're relieved that by conducting this "experiment" you proved that chocolate doesn't give you headaches. Sorry. This was not a scientific experiment. A scientific experiment focuses on a single, isolated variable, but there are always *multiple* triggers—a complex, ever-changing mixture—stacking up against your threshold for activation of migraine. These background triggers are not only unavoidable but also difficult to monitor. It would be handy if you had a gauge that could tell you whether your trigger level stands at 5 percent, or 50 percent, or 95 percent of your threshold, and thereby know how careful you have to be, but you don't. Not knowing where your background trigger level stands is all the more reason to avoid adding the dietary items that just might raise it above your threshold.

The fact is that for many people chocolate and many other dietary triggers always *contribute* to the likelihood of a headache, even if they don't always *cause* a headache—depending on the load of other triggers that you're carrying to begin with. But for the reasons described above, headache sufferers often convince themselves of what they want to believe: that certain dietary triggers (which they love to eat) don't play an important role, since the role they play seems inconsistent. Know anyone like that?

Even worse, caffeine—one of the most potent dietary triggers—has a paradoxical effect that makes it appear *helpful* for headaches in the short run even though it *increases* headaches in the long run. This is true of caffeine-containing beverages including coffee, tea (and iced tea) and certain sodas such as colas, Mountain Dew and Dr Pepper. The reason is that caffeine constricts blood vessels. If blood vessels around your head are painfully swollen because of migraine, and therefore you have a headache, caffeine may provide temporary relief by constricting the vessels. This is why many headache sufferers, recognizing that a strong cup

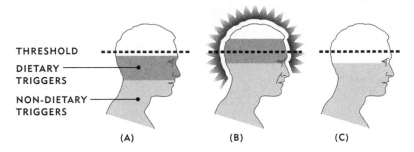

THRESHOLD
DIETARY TRIGGERS
NON-DIETARY TRIGGERS

(A)   (B)   (C)

FIGURE 7: WHY DIETARY TRIGGERS MATTER. *Before symptoms appear, dietary triggers are present but inconsequential (A). With a rise in nondietary triggers (B), symptoms occur because the total trigger level exceeds the threshold. Eliminating dietary triggers reduces the level (C), and symptoms are again controlled.*

of coffee or a Coke may ward off an impending headache, gravitate toward dietary caffeine. It's also why caffeine is an ingredient in Excedrin, Fiorinal and Fioricet, and other quick-fix medications for headaches.

The problem is that as caffeine and its constricting influence wear off, rebound vasodilation—increased blood vessel swelling—occurs. (This is why people get headaches when they don't have their usual caffeine fix early in the morning or when they try cutting back on caffeine intake.) The occurrence of rebound vasodilation when the constricting influence of caffeine wears off is the reason caffeine *contributes* to headaches long-term. But because you may initially feel relief, you fail to realize that caffeine ultimately worsens your headaches and therefore must be eliminated.

Another reason for confusion about dietary triggers for migraine is that *not* eating on schedule—that is, skipping or delaying meals—can be a trigger. If you don't eat breakfast and lunch, and get a whopping headache as a result, you may think, *Well, I sure don't get my headaches from food!* If that's what you think, you're overlooking the multifactor-

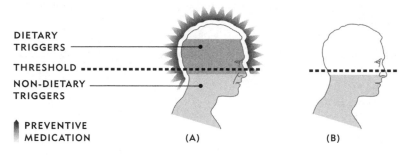

FIGURE 8: DIETARY MODIFICATION. *Before dietary modification, migraine symptoms are active (A). In this case, eliminating dietary triggers is sufficient to bring the total trigger level below the threshold (B), and symptoms are controlled.*

ial way in which your headaches are triggered—and you're overlooking opportunities to reduce your exposure to certain key, avoidable triggers.

Some headache sufferers fail to recognize the full extent of their dietary triggers because their headaches are so chronic. If you always, or almost always, *already* have a headache, it's hard to recognize anything that's causing or contributing to having a headache.

You might say, *But I didn't change my diet when I started getting headaches, so it can't be my diet.* No, it's not *just* your diet, but it's partly your diet. You'd been carrying a load of dietary triggers all along, but until something else changed—a fall in your threshold or a rise in some other trigger(s)—it didn't matter. But now that you're having headaches it does matter, and you can do something about the situation: *possibly* by dealing with whatever else changed, but *definitely* by avoiding the dietary items that formerly were inconsequential but now are part of the problem (see Figure 7, page 69).

Many of my new headache patients tell me they've tried dietary modification without success in the past, and that has reinforced their belief that dietary triggers aren't important. Rarely did they do dietary

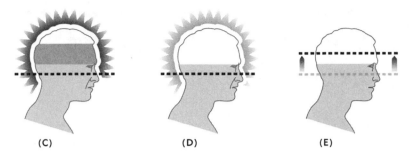

(C)   (D)   (E)

In this scenario, before dietary modification the trigger level is high and symptoms are active (C). In this case, dietary triggers must be eliminated to reduce the total level, even though it may remain above the threshold (D). Preventive medication can then raise the threshold (E) so that symptoms are controlled.

modification properly, as I'm about to explain. Usually, prior trials have eliminated at most a few items at a time, and only for a short time. That's not good enough.

And even when dietary modification is done properly but fails to control headaches satisfactorily, this doesn't mean that dietary triggers aren't important. All it means is that dietary modification alone may not be sufficient to lower your total trigger level below your threshold. Dietary modification is nonetheless necessary in order for additional actions—potentially including Step 3, preventive medication—to achieve the goal of a subthreshold trigger level (see Figure 8, above). But let's not get too far ahead of ourselves; first let's look carefully at the ins and outs of dietary control of headaches.

Eliminating Dietary Triggers

EVERYONE'S DIFFERENT, and it may be that not every one of the foods and beverages that most commonly cause headaches is a trigger for you, but the items that appear in Table 6 (pages 74–75) are the common cul-

Why Most Doctors Don't Believe in the Migraine Diet

The impression of most doctors that dietary modification doesn't work to control headaches is based in part on misunderstanding and in part on misuse of the dietary approach. Doctors generally share their patients' failure to recognize the important role of dietary triggers and are therefore unequipped to educate patients properly.

Proper education is essential in order to guide and motivate you to do the right things with your diet and thereby help control your headaches. For instance, if a doctor gives you a list of potential dietary triggers but doesn't explain *why* you haven't recognized them, you're likely to respond (silently): *What, you think I'm stupid? Like I wouldn't have figured this out for myself if it were true?* And then you're not going to follow the diet.

Doctors who do address dietary issues in headache treatment too often advise patients to eliminate one item at a time, which rarely works. It is unlikely that eliminating any one dietary trigger alone will reduce your total trigger level below your threshold. Still worse, doctors tend to half-heartedly introduce dietary modification as an offhand, semi-pointless effort, accompanied by the explanation, or at least the attitude: *Well, I'm not sure that this will do any good . . .*

Guess what happens? It's yet another example of how low expectations preordain headache treatment failure. ◆

---

prits. You can begin to take control of your headaches by eliminating *each and every one* of these potential triggers from your diet. (Later, you may be able to reintroduce some of these foods and beverages, as I'll explain, but for now strict compliance is required.)

The better you follow the diet, the more likely you are to achieve headache control, and the less likely it is that you will require preventive medication—or the less preventive medication you will require—in order to achieve headache control. No one can follow the diet perfectly, *but do your best*. Each dietary trigger you avoid, thereby removing it from your stack of triggers, reduces your total trigger level and increases the likelihood that you can keep the level below your threshold. Remember, since there are so many triggers that are unavoidable, or difficult or undesirable to avoid (see Table 5, page 62), it is all the more important to eliminate the potent but generally unrecognized triggers that you *can* avoid readily: the dietary items (and medications) detailed in this chapter.

The diet is a tool. The more skillfully you use any tool, the better it will function. The better you use this tool, the diet, the more effective it will be in controlling your headaches. If your goal is to control your headaches—and take as little medication as possible—the diet is the most valuable tool you have.

You might criticize the diet for its "negative" approach, and it's true that it focuses on what you cannot eat and drink rather than on what you can. But the number of items you *are* allowed to eat and drink is much greater than what you're not, and listing them would require too much space. And just in case you need some help, you'll find some sample menus and recipes and other dietary tips in the Appendix. (Don't be constrained by these suggestions; they're just examples to get you started.)

The diet can be tough to follow initially, especially for vegetarians and others on already restricted diets, but it is *not* a life sentence of culinary deprivation. Cheer up: you can look forward to a time when your headaches have been controlled well enough, long enough that you can afford to rock the boat by carefully experimenting with dietary liberalization. It's likely that eventually you can tolerate some of the initially restricted items, at least in limited quantities. But at the start you must strictly avoid *all* potential dietary triggers. Dietary liberalization comes

Dietary Triggers

CAFFEINE	Coffee, tea, iced tea and cola. Even decaf coffee and tea (which contain additional chemical triggers) may be a problem. Also, beware of coffee substitutes. Try caffeine-free herb tea (without citrus and other trigger flavors).
CHOCOLATE	White chocolate is okay; I'm not so sure about carob.
MONOSODIUM GLUTAMATE	Chinese (and other) restaurant food; soups and bouillons; Accent and seasoned salt; flavored, salty snacks; croutons and bread crumbs; gravies; ready-to-eat meals; cheap buffets; processed meats; veggie burgers; protein concentrates; and low-fat, low-calorie foods. Watch out for hidden MSG (see Table 7, page 81).
PROCESSED MEATS AND FISH	Aged, canned, cured, fermented, marinated, smoked, tenderized—or preserved with nitrites or nitrates. Hot dogs, sausage, salami, pepperoni, bologna (and other lunchmeats with nitrites), liverwurst, beef jerky, certain hams, bacon, pâtés, smoked or pickled fish, caviar and anchovies. Also, fresh beef liver and chicken livers, and wild game (which contain tyramine).
CHEESE AND OTHER DAIRY PRODUCTS	The more aged, the worse. (Permissible cheeses include cottage cheese, ricotta, cream cheese and good-quality American cheese.) Beware of cheese-containing foods, including pizza. Yogurt (including frozen yogurt), sour cream and buttermilk are also triggers.
NUTS	Avoid all kinds, as well as nut butters. Seeds are okay.
ALCOHOL AND VINEGAR	Especially red wine, champagne and dark or heavy drinks. Vodka is best tolerated. Clear (ideally, distilled) vinegar is *allowable*. Don't overdo condiments (ketchup, mustard and mayonnaise) made with vinegar.
CERTAIN FRUITS AND JUICES	Citrus fruits (oranges, grapefruits, lemons, limes, tanger-ines, clementines and pineapples) and their juices—as well as bananas. Also avoid raisins (and other dried fruits if preserved with sulfites), raspberries, red plums, papayas, passion fruit, figs, dates and avocados.
CERTAIN VEGETABLES, ESPECIALLY ONIONS	Plus sauerkraut, pea pods and certain beans (broad Italian, lima, fava, and navy, and lentils). *Allowed:* leeks, scallions, shallots, spring onions; also garlic.

Table 6

Dietary Triggers (continued)

FRESH YEAST-RISEN BAKED GOODS	Less than one day old: homemade (or restaurant-baked) breads, especially sourdough, as well as bagels, doughnuts, pizza dough, soft pretzels and coffee cake.
ASPARTAME (NUTRASWEET)	Saccharin (Sweet'n Low) may also be a trigger for some. As far as I know, sucralose (Splenda) isn't a problem.
OTHERS?	Perhaps soy products, especially if cultured (miso), fermented (tempeh) or otherwise highly processed (e.g., soy protein isolate/concentrate). Watch out for soy sauce containing MSG. Less risky are unflavored tofu and soy milk and flour. Soy oil is safe. Possibly tomatoes (and tomato-based sauces), mushrooms . . . whatever gives *you* a headache.

Table 6

only *after* you have achieved headache control and maintained it for four months or more. The details of how you can attempt to reintroduce items will be spelled out later in this chapter.

When Is a Dietary Item a Migraine Trigger?

ANY RESEMBLANCE OF MIGRAINE dietary triggers to food allergies is only superficial. The role of dietary triggers in migraine has nothing to do with allergy, which is when your body's immune (defense) system overreacts to something. The effect of dietary triggers in migraine is not mediated by the immune system.

Having said that, I have to admit that the specific way in which dietary items trigger migraine is unclear. I find it helpful to imagine that they directly feed into and stimulate the migraine control center in the brain, stacking with other, nondietary triggers such as stress, hormones and barometric pressure changes, and pushing your total trigger level toward (or farther above) your threshold. The effect of each dietary trigger is dose-related: the more, the worse.

Want to Lose Weight?

Many people who follow the migraine-preventive diet are pleased with the results: fewer headaches as well as fewer pounds to bear.

But be careful about other weight-loss measures. Cutting fat and calories is fine; so is exercise. It's the diet pills and supplements that I worry about. Diet pills, whether prescription, over-the-counter or herbal, contain chemicals that may suppress your appetite or boost your metabolism but in the process trigger migraine. Diet supplements, including protein drinks (canned or powdered), low-carbohydrate energy bars and frozen diet meals, are often headache bombs full of explosive MSG.

Don't fret. If you just eat right—and exercise properly—you can control your headaches *and* shed weight. ◆

No single chemical trigger is common among all the dietary items on the list. Quite a number of chemicals can be problematic—caffeine, monosodium glutamate, nitrites and nitrates, tyramine, alcohols and aspartame, among others—and different ones are contained in the various foods and beverages listed.

Caffeine

CAFFEINATED BEVERAGES—coffee, tea, iced tea, chocolate drinks, cola and other caffeine-containing sodas—should be eliminated completely and permanently. Elimination of caffeine may be associated with withdrawal symptoms, including increased headaches, for up to a few weeks. If rebound resulting from quick-fix medications is also a problem that must be eliminated, you might as well get rid of caffeine and the quick fixes at the same time; it's best to get over whatever increased headaches may result as soon as possible.

I recommend cold-turkeying dietary caffeine. The alternative is a quick taper—to *zero*—within no more than two weeks. Tapering has the potential advantage of lessening whatever withdrawal headaches you may have, but this is outweighed by the disadvantage of dragging out the process so that, despite your best intentions, it never reaches its end.

Decaffeinated coffee and tea contain chemicals other than caffeine (a small amount

Who Says They're Triggers?

The recognition of certain dietary items as triggers is based on cumulative experience among headache sufferers. Scientific studies have shed little light on dietary triggers for migraine, in part because it's impossible to isolate individual dietary items for study while maintaining a steady-state background of other, uncontrollable triggers and in part because no single factor *always* triggers migraine.

The failure of most of the few scientific studies that have looked at migraine dietary triggers to demonstrate a clear effect is a good example of the limitations of science in identifying truth that is otherwise obvious. Try telling a headache sufferer who has had killer headaches after eating chocolate or drinking red wine that it's all in his or her imagination!

Still, I occasionally wonder if *all* of these dietary items belong on this list. A number of times, just when I've been about to scratch one off to make things simpler, patients have come back and told me that they've reintroduced certain dietary items (without recurrent headaches) *except* the item in question, which for them is a clear trigger. And so the list has endured more or less intact over the years. ✦

of which remains after decaffeination) that can be triggers. So, ideally, even decaffeinated coffee and tea should be avoided. But if the only way you can stop drinking regular coffee or tea is to switch to decaf, well, that's better than continuing to consume regular coffee or tea.

Caffeine-free herb teas, on the other hand, pose no problem—as long as they don't contain too many other triggering flavors such as citrus, raisin or pineapple—and are the best substitute if you want a warm beverage. Don't be fooled into thinking that green tea is caffeine-free: it's not, by a long shot. Caffeine-*free* beverages (that is, those without caffeine in the first place) such as caffeine-free cola are fine, but you

Coffee Substitutes?

These beverages, typically made from chicory and carob, make me nervous. They're often flavored with an assortment of migraine triggers, including orange peel, figs and almonds, and malted barley—a potential MSG source—is found in most of these products.

Stick with herbal tea until you've achieved control of your head- aches. Then maybe you can begin to experiment with some of the coffee substitutes. ◆

should stay away from diet sodas containing NutraSweet (aspartame), which also can be a trigger.

You may argue that you can't give up caf- feine because you need it to get started in the morning and keep going through the day; you feel so tired as it is, and you can't imagine life without it. If so, you're overlooking the roller coaster effect of caffeine. After each rise comes a fall in energy for which you feel the need for another cup of coffee, which leads to the next fall, and so on. Most people who can't imag- ine living without caffeine feel *much better* in general—with improved energy, sounder sleep, less irritability, reduced heartburn and fewer palpitations, not to mention decreased headaches—after eliminating caffeine and getting through a few weeks of withdrawal, which may not even be noticeable.

Chocolate

IT FIGURES THAT anything as sinfully delicious as chocolate would be sinful when it comes to migraine. It's not just that chocolate (and anything made with chocolate or cocoa) contains caffeine; it has other migraine- triggering chemicals, including theobromine and phenylethylamine. White chocolate is safe, but carob-containing items make me uneasy: maybe they're okay, but I haven't learned to trust them.

Chocolate: Illusion or Trigger?

It has been suggested that the association between chocolate and headaches is not a cause-and-effect relationship, but an illusion. From this point of view, for example, an impending menstrual period produces not only craving for (and indulgence in) chocolate but also headache—because of the period, not the chocolate. Chocolate and headache thereby become associated, and causation is assumed. This point of view is partly a response to a few studies that have failed to show consistent triggering of migraine in response to chocolate.

As I've already explained, it's not surprising that these studies have been negative.

Migraine dietary triggers don't act in isolation; they act in concert with other, fluctuating trigger factors that are difficult to identify and control. There's no doubt in my mind—or in the minds of thousands of headache sufferers—that chocolate and the other items on the list are triggers for many, if not most people. It's laughable to insist otherwise, as do some doctors who bow to (misleading) scientific data rather than listening to what their patients have to say, loudly and clearly. The last time I checked, none of my *male* headache patients was having chocolate cravings around *his* periods, but a lot of these guys have no doubt that chocolate spells trouble . . . all month long. ◆

You can satisfy your sweet tooth with just about everything other than chocolate—including caramel and sugary treats of all kinds—although some people find licorice to be a trigger, too.

Monosodium Glutamate

YOU MAY BE FAMILIAR with the common presence of monosodium glutamate (MSG) in Chinese restaurant food. You may not realize that MSG is nearly *everywhere* and often *hidden behind other names*. The names of substances that contain MSG and are ingredients in many prepared foods appear in Table 7 (page 81). (Monosodium glutamate is considered "natural" by the U.S. Food and Drug Administration and may even be present in foods whose labels proclaim "all natural" and "no artificial ingredients.") Avoiding MSG is the trickiest challenge in following the migraine-preventive diet.

If you read labels carefully, you'll discover that many commercially prepared foods—those that are processed and then canned, jarred, bottled, bagged, boxed or frozen—contain either MSG itself or an ingredient rich in MSG. The effect of MSG is to create or enhance

"I couldn't imagine life without coffee"

PAUL'S STORY

A self-admitted "java junkie," Paul was opposed to giving up what he considered to be one of life's greatest pleasures. But he also didn't like having "background" headaches every day, and debilitating headaches several times a month, so he agreed to sacrifice caffeine and see what would happen.

It wasn't easy for the first week or so; he was in bed for several days with "a killer." But his headaches quickly subsided and he was surprised how much better he felt all over. Instead of feeling more tired, he became more energetic and slept much better. He also had a lot fewer aches and pains throughout his body—not to mention no more heartburn from reflux!

Paul was careful about the complete diet at first, but he gradually reintroduced every one of the restricted items—except caffeine—without recurrent headaches. For him, as for many of my patients, caffeine turned out to be the primary dietary culprit. ◆

Potential Sources of MSG

Hydrolyzed* protein (including vegetable/ soy/plant/rice protein)	Textured protein	Sodium or calcium caseinate
	Whey protein	
		Glutamic acid
Yeast extract and autolyzed yeast	Protein-fortified items	
		Gelatin
	Malt extract	
Natural flavors/ flavorings		Fermented or cultured items
	Malted barley	
Broth, stock or bouillon	Maltodextrin	Ultra-pasteurized items
	Carrageenan	Enzyme-modified items
Soy protein concentrate/isolate	Kombu (seaweed extract)	

*The term "hydrogenated" does *not* signify MSG.

Note: Also beware of similar-sounding items.

Table 7

savory flavor, so it helps to restore flavor that is lost in the process of commercial food preparation. (Savory flavor—umami—is a brothy, meaty sensation that has been called the "fifth" basic taste, in addition to salt, sweet, sour and bitter. Some even claim that MSG is the *sole* chemical stimulus of umami and can't imagine where we'd be without the pleasure it gives us!) Especially MSG-laden are soups and bouillons; Accent and seasoned salt; flavored, salty snacks; croutons and bread crumbs; gravies; ready-to-eat meals; cheap buffets; processed meats; veggie burgers; protein concentrates; and low-fat, low-calorie foods (to which MSG is added to compensate for the reduced content of yummy fat and sugar).

When an ingredient list includes "natural flavors (or flavorings)," be especially suspicious that means MSG when the food item is more savory (or salty) than sweet. And be aware that although ingredient

What Is MSG?

Let's start with glutamic acid, one of the amino acids that are the building blocks of proteins. It's present throughout our bodies, including our brains, where in its "free" form—unbound to protein—it acts as an excitatory neurotransmitter. In addition, not only proteins containing glutamic acid but also free glutamate are naturally present in much of what we eat and drink.

MSG—monosodium glutamate—is the free salt form of glutamic acid. It's usually produced by fermentation of molasses made from sugar beet or sugarcane. But it seems that *processed* free glutamate, arising from vegetable protein breakdown in commercial food preparation, behaves badly—unlike *natural* free glutamate. Whether or not that's the right explanation, something in foods containing MSG sure behaves badly when it comes to migraine. ◆

lists are ordered according to the relative amounts of each ingredient, MSG (and MSG-laden surrogates such as hydrolyzed protein) are *very potent triggers*. Even a small amount, meriting placement near the end of a list of many other ingredients, may cause major migraine problems.

Watch out for tuna packed in water or oil containing hydrolyzed protein; you *may* be able to get away with it if you squeeze out the water or oil well enough. Or, if you look around—at organic-oriented markets, for instance—you can find tuna *not* packed with hydrolyzed protein. The same is true of sausages: some have MSG (usually labeled overtly as such) with or without nitrites, and some don't. *The best way to avoid MSG is to eat food made from fresh ingredients.* Otherwise, *read labels carefully.*

Many restaurants routinely use MSG or MSG-containing ingredients in their kitchens. Even when restaurants claim to be MSG-free, be forewarned: they may not sprinkle MSG powder directly into their food, but they may use MSG-containing ingredients without realizing it. The simpler the food preparation, the better; you're most likely to get into trouble with sauces, casseroles, soups and seasoned coatings. And watch out for fast food that's fortified with MSG (whether identified as such or under an alias) to overcome its mass-produced blandness . . . especially seasoned fries, breading on chicken and fish, and "special sauces."

Processed Meats and Fish

MEATS AND FISH that are aged, canned, cured, fermented, marinated, smoked or tenderized—or preserved with nitrites or nitrates—are common dietary triggers of migraine. Beware of hot dogs, sausages (not all contain nitrites but may have MSG *and* tyramine, another powerful trigger), salami, pepperoni, bologna (and other lunch meats with nitrites), liverwurst, beef jerky, certain hams, bacon and pâtés, as well as smoked salmon or trout, caviar, anchovies and pickled fish (such as herring). *Ask questions* about nitrites and nitrates at the deli counter; the server can check labels for you. Be aware that some *un*processed meats, such as beef and chicken livers and wild game, are also high in tyramine.

A general rule: tyramine (along with glutamate) tends to accumulate with aging and ripening. In avoiding foods that trigger migraine, *young and fresh is best.*

You'll often find thiamine mono*nitrate* listed as an ingredient in enriched flour; I think it's okay—not a trigger. More and more, specialty grocery stores offer items without nitrites and nitrates (and with less MSG).

Cheese and Other Dairy Products

TYRAMINE IS ALSO THE CULPRIT here and is especially abundant in aged cheeses. If you crave cheese, try young cheeses that are relatively low in tyramine: cottage cheese, ricotta, cream cheese and good-quality American cheese. After controlling your headaches well enough and long enough to be able to risk rocking your boat, you might try adding back other relatively young cheeses, such as fresh goat cheese, or mozzarella.

Food Fight on the Web!

In one corner we have the MSG-phobes, who claim that MSG causes a whole lot of what ails us: *www.msg myth.com*; *www.nomsg.com*; and *www.truthinlabeling.org*

In the other corner stand MSG manufacturers and the food industry, who want us to be grateful for the ways in which MSG enhances the flavor of our food: *www.msg.org* and *www.ajinomoto-malaysia.com*.

Refereeing (though some would say in the pockets of the food establishment) are "neutral" parties such as the FDA: *www.fda.gov*.

In dispute is what is (or isn't) MSG and what it can (or can't)

do to you. I don't accept everything the MSG-phobes claim, but I believe they're on to something, at least when it comes to headaches. You can check it out for yourself, but trust me: *if you have headaches, avoid MSG.*

The pro-MSG advocates' position—that MSG is totally benign and beneficial—is full of holes. Excuse me, but I've heard too many patients describe misery induced by eating Chinese restaurant food—or soups, or snack items like Doritos—and had too many similar experiences myself to *not* know when I'm being hit on the head with a hammer. ◆

But watch out for cheese-containing foods such as pizza, which can be a double, triple or quadruple whammy on account of not only cheese but also ingredients in the sauce, toppings (pepperoni, sausage, onions and canned items soaked in MSG) and yeast-risen dough.

Other dairy products—yogurt (including frozen yogurt), sour cream and buttermilk—can trigger migraine. Milk, cream, butter and ice cream are usually not a problem. (The "ice cream headaches" caused by eating ice cream or some other very cold item too quickly are variations of migraine but are triggered by temperature, not by chemical components.)

Nuts

NUTS IN GENERAL—pistachios, walnuts, cashews, Brazil nuts, pecans, almonds, coconuts—as well as nut butters and extracts contain tyramine and are therefore potential migraine triggers. Peanuts (which are actually legumes) and peanut butter should also be avoided. Seeds, such as sunflower and pumpkin seeds, are not a problem.

Alcohol and Vinegar

ALCOHOLIC BEVERAGES can trigger migraine in several ways. Too much alcohol at once leads to accumulation of acetaldehydes (breakdown products of alcohol), which trigger the migraine experience known as a hangover. (Yes, a hangover is migraine.) Another way relates to congeners, chemicals that develop in the process of fermenting certain alcoholic beverages, especially red wine, cognac and other dark liqueurs, spirits, and sparkling wines including champagne. Congeners are what give these drinks their distinctive characteristics, but they're also largely why you're more prone to headaches after drinking them rather than, for example, white wine.

Among alcoholic beverages, vodka—which is low in congeners—is best tolerated in limited quantities. You might find that specific wines or beers are okay, while others—even of generally similar type—aren't. Sulfites, trig-

Spice It Up!

Other than seasoning mixtures containing MSG, you needn't fear the contents of your spice rack. Instead, get friendly with herbs and spices, and use them to liven up the foods you're allowed on the migraine-preventive diet. You should restrict certain items from your plate (Table 6, pages 74–75), but you can still indulge your palate.

Be bold and have fun: aside from the usual array of flavorings, including all kinds of peppers (and peppercorns) and garlic, consider curries, ginger, horseradish, mustard seed and powder, cardamom, cinnamon, mint, vanilla, honey . . . you get the picture. ◆

gers for some people, are part of the problem with certain wines causing headaches, as are phenols. Both wine and beer (even "nonalcoholic") also contain tyramine and other, related vasoactive (migraine-triggering) amines. Some tap (draft) beers may be higher in tyramine—and consequently in its migraine-triggering action—than bottled ones.

Vinegars are also fermentation products, and dark ones (especially balsamic, which contains sulfites) should be avoided, but clear white vinegar—ideally, distilled—is permissible. Be careful not to overdo condiments (ketchup, mustard and mayonnaise) and pickled products that are prepared with vinegar; if you have a choice, you're better off with those made with distilled (rather than apple cider) vinegar.

Certain Fruits and Juices

CITRUS FRUITS (oranges, grapefruits, lemons, limes, tangerines, clementines, pineapples) and their juices are healthful foods in so many respects that it may seem odd to include them in a list of items to avoid. Don't be fooled: these stealth triggers are potent troublemakers for many headache sufferers. Vitamin C is no problem. (In fact, it's a good idea to take a high-potency multivitamin daily while following the migraine-preventive diet.) Citric acid is also permissible.

Bananas are, for many, a *big* trigger. Raisins, other dried fruits (if preserved with sulfites), raspberries, red plums, papayas, passion fruit, figs, dates and avocados (including guacamole) are also relatively high in tyramine. I'd always thought kiwis were no problem . . . until an especially thoughtful, observant patient informed me that kiwis are a *major* trigger for her. I still tend to think that they're okay in general and that this is a good example of varying individual sensitivity to certain items—and why you need to keep a lookout for yourself. Or maybe her kiwis were just overripe.

Before you start to think that there's no fruit left for you to enjoy without fear of headaches, hold on: help yourself to apples, most berries, cherries, grapes, melons, peaches, pears and more, as spelled out in the Appendix (see page 221).

Certain Vegetables, Especially Onions

BESIDES ONIONS (and onion powder), this category includes sauerkraut, pea pods and certain beans (containing tyramine): broad Italian, lima, fava and navy, as well as lentils. After you have controlled your headaches, if you wish to experiment with reintroducing potential dietary triggers, you may find that you can tolerate cooked onions better than raw ones. Leeks, scallions, shallots, and spring onions are safe. So is garlic.

Fresh Yeast-Risen Baked Goods

WATCH OUT FOR fresh (less than one day old) homemade (or restaurant-baked) breads, especially sourdough, as well as other fresh-baked, yeast-risen bakery items including bagels, doughnuts, pizza dough, soft pretzels and coffee cake. This category is an exception to the rule that fresher is better when it comes to avoiding migraine. Instead, packaged commercial breads from a supermarket are less likely to contribute to headaches than home-baked bread right out of the oven. Don't forget to stay away from baked goods containing cheese, nuts, chocolate, bananas, raisins, citrus and other such triggers. And be careful about croutons and packaged bread crumbs that are "seasoned" . . . with MSG.

Aspartame (NutraSweet)

WHILE ASPARTAME IS a clear-cut migraine trigger factor for some individuals, certain other artificial sweeteners—such as sorbitol, xylitol, mannitol and sucralose (Splenda)—and sugar itself generally don't stimulate headaches. (I've had a few patients whose headaches have decreased dramatically just by eliminating diet sodas with aspartame. If you're looking for a caffeine-free diet cola without aspartame, try Diet Rite, which contains sucralose rather than aspartame.) Saccharin

Oh, Ye of Little Faith

Have you noticed how those closest to you seem to listen to you least? Well, that was true of my beloved secretary, Carolyn. After years of answering my patients' questions about the diet and witnessing their remarkable responses to dietary modification, Carolyn *still* didn't quite get it. When she complained to me one day of jaw pain, I asked her what she'd had to eat earlier. Wouldn't you know: a *banana*. Carolyn was unconvinced, but after a few more banana-induced jaw pains she conceded that I was right.

P.S.: When Carolyn's sister Clara heard about this, she admitted to feeling "on the verge of something bad" when *she* eats a banana. I suppose one difference between the two sisters' reactions is that Carolyn carries the additional trigger load of working with me. ◆

(Sweet'n Low) is said by some to be a problem at times, but I haven't seen that in my practice.

Other Dietary Items

YOU MAY RECOGNIZE personal dietary triggers that aren't on the list. For instance, tomatoes and tomato-based sauces are triggers for some people—perhaps because tomatoes naturally contain relatively high levels of free glutamate. Mushrooms and peas, too. Some people feel they have problems with wheat, milk or pork. The list of restrictions is long enough as it is, and adding more items would make adherence to it even more daunting—and compliance less likely. If you suspect other dietary triggers, by all means avoid them.

Let's Catch Our Breath

IN CASE YOU'RE STILL feeling resistant, let me reassure you of two things: (1) you *can* control your headaches, either with the diet alone or in part with the help of the diet, and (2) once you've controlled your headaches, you'll be able to liberalize the diet to some degree. More about this at the end of this chapter, but I thought it might help to dangle a carrot (which, by the way, you can eat all you want). Now let's look at some other avoidable, but nondietary triggers.

What About Soy?

The truth is, I'm not exactly sure. You won't find tofu, soy sauce or other soy products on my list of items to avoid, but they often appear on other, similar lists. It's the single dietary issue I've struggled with the most, going back and forth in my mind as I wander up and down supermarket aisles and listen to patients' observations in my office, trying to decide whether these items are trouble or not.

Soy sauce contains tyramine, and some soy sauces also list MSG; these are both ingredients to be avoided. Watch out for miso and the fermented soybean cake called tempeh, both of which are prepared by processes involving hydrolysis (breakdown) of soy protein, which liberates MSG. Soy burgers are usually *loaded* with MSG (without which they wouldn't taste like much). I also worry about dietary protein supplements—liquid mixtures, powders and low-carbohydrate energy bars— that contain soy protein concentrate (or isolate). Stay away from these highly processed (or "refined") soy derivatives; you *may* be relatively safe with the more natural, straightforward items such as soy milk (but not cheese or yogurt), soy flour and tofu (as long as it's not flavored with some other culprit). As far as I can figure, soy oil is safe. But even plain old soybeans contain tyramine.

Soy isoflavones are so-called phytoestrogens (plant estrogens) taken in tablet form for their alleged estrogen-like effects. I haven't noticed any obvious problem among my migraine patients doing so, at least not yet. But if these substances really act like estrogen, then it wouldn't surprise me. If you do consume soy in one form or another and can't get rid of your head-aches, or you try a soy product and your headaches worsen, don't be surprised . . . and do avoid it. ◆

Medication Triggers

THE OTHER CATEGORY of migraine triggers that are swallowed and can be avoided is medications. I am referring not to the quick fixes that cause rebound, but rather to medications that directly stimulate the migraine control center (see Table 8, page 91). In some cases these medications are optional and therefore avoidable, and in other cases they may be mandatory and unavoidable. You should always communicate with your prescribing doctor before you eliminate any prescription medication.

As with dietary items, the role these medications play in triggering migraine may not be obvious, for a number of reasons. Especially with birth-control pills and hormone replacement therapy, you may begin experiencing headaches *months after* starting the medication. This delay reduces the likelihood that you'll recognize the link and provides grounds for doubting a connection should you even consider the possibility.

In addition, when a medication such as birth-control pills serves one or more useful purposes, your benefit from the medication may encourage you to deny that it's contributing to your headaches. Or, you may try to eliminate birth-control pills (or some other medication suspected of contributing to headaches) for a few months without seeing improvement, as a result of which you may conclude that the medication is not a trigger.

You may be wrong. Remember: as with dietary items, the elimination of medications that add to your total trigger level may or may not be sufficient to achieve a subthreshold trigger level, but may nonetheless be a *necessary* step—which needs to be combined with other steps if you're to reach the goal.

You have to decide for yourself whether a medication that potentially triggers migraine—and is not *essential* for whatever purpose you take it—is worth eliminating or not. It's a cost-benefit analysis: weigh-

Medication Triggers

HORMONES	Hormonal contraception, including birth-control pills, medroxy-progesterone injections (Depo-Provera) and levonorgestrel implants (Norplant)
	Hormone replacement therapy
	Other hormonal treatments
ADRENALINE-LIKE DRUGS, STIMULANTS AND DIET PILLS	Bronchodilators for asthma (e.g., Proventil, Serevent)
	Over-the-counter stimulants (e.g., No-Doz), including herbal stimulants
	Methylphenidate (Ritalin, Concerta)
	Dextroamphetamine (Adderall, Dexedrine)
	Over-the-counter diet pills
	Prescription diet pills (e.g., Ionamin, Meridia)
VASODILATORS	Nitrates for heart disease (e.g., Isordil, Nitro-Dur)
	Sildenafil citrate (Viagra)
OTHERS	Isotretinoin (Accutane) for acne
	Selective serotonin reuptake inhibitors (e.g., Prozac) and buproprion (Wellbutrin) for depression

Table 8

ing the intended virtues of the medication against the potential for better headache control by eliminating it.

From a headache perspective, the best approach is to eliminate nonessential medication that may be contributing to headaches, thereby achieving headache control (also using whatever other steps you may need to take), and decide later whether to try adding back the medication. You may or may not be able to add it back without suffering recurrent headaches, but at least in that setting—*after* you've achieved headache control—you can more clearly assess the contribution (or lack thereof) of that medication to your headaches.

While some medications listed as triggers may be deemed essential because they're being taken for potentially serious medical problems including asthma and heart disease, there may be treatment alternatives that would work as well or better yet wouldn't trigger migraine. This is especially true in the case of asthma, for which non-triggering medication options abound. If you're taking one of the medications listed, you should discuss alternatives with your treating doctor.

"Sometimes it takes a while"

CATHY'S STORY

I t took several visits for me to get through to Cathy. She really didn't want to follow the diet, partly because she was very skeptical and partly because she felt overwhelmed by other concerns, like worrying about periods of forgetfulness and the possibility that she had Alzheimer's disease (which she didn't).

Finally, Cathy bought into the diet, and she's done, in her word, "great" for the past four years. She mentioned to me last visit that she thinks it would take anyone at least a couple of months to really learn how to follow the diet properly, and maybe a couple more months to benefit maximally. So keep Cathy's perspective in mind as you go forward.

Oh, by the way: Cathy no longer feels so forgetful, now that her headaches are controlled, and she's stopped worrying about Alzheimer's disease. She's also successfully reintroduced yogurt and decaf coffee, although she had major headaches when she tried orange juice, bananas and cheese. ◆

Other medications not listed in Table 8 may be a trigger for some people, including you. For sure, some medications given to prevent rejection after organ transplant can provoke headaches. From time to time I've wondered about others: for instance, omeprazole (Prilosec) and other proton pump inhibitors for gastroesophageal reflux, and drugs for elevated cholesterol (the "statins"). I'm just not sure—at least not sure enough to list them. But pay attention to your own experience with these or any other drugs and decide for yourself.

Hormonal Contraception

IF YOU'RE ON HORMONAL CONTRACEPTION such as birth-control pills, Depo-Provera or Norplant for birth-control purposes only, and if headaches are a problem, talk with your doctor about switching to an alternative, nonhormonal form of birth control. Hormonal contraceptives are potent migraine triggers for many women, although recognition of this often is obscured. There may not be a noticeable increase in headaches when you start hormonal contraception, if *without* the drug your total trigger level is *already* far above your threshold. Hormonal contraception nonetheless becomes a further contributor to your total stack of triggers, making it that much harder to reduce the level below your threshold.

Step by Step

If you wanted to walk through a doorway 10 feet away, you would need to take at least several steps. Imagine this: taking a single step; deciding that because you haven't yet reached the doorway, that step isn't worthwhile; backstepping to where you started; and repeating this cycle over and over, one insufficient step at a time, never adding up to an effective *series* of steps to reach your goal.

It wouldn't make sense. Yet people do this all the time in trying to control their headaches. They take one step at a time and backstep after each one, since each alone didn't control their headaches. Whether or not certain steps are by themselves *sufficient* to control your headaches, they may nonetheless be *necessary*, and in the right combination, they will be sufficient. ◆

Occasionally, hormonal contraception is prescribed to prevent headaches. Sometimes cyclical therapy is used, in which case menstrual periods occur, and sometimes treatment is continuous, usually with the intention of suppressing menses and avoiding menstrual headaches. Or, estrogen may just be given temporarily around the time of menstruation in order to smooth out the normal dip in estrogen levels at

---

"You mean I just needed to get off birth-control pills?"

≋

ROBERTA'S STORY

R oberta never needed a brain MRI scan. It was obvious, at least to me, that her headaches were due to migraine. But before I saw her a scan had been done, and it showed a small vascular malformation: a benign tangle of blood vessels in her brain.

This malformation had nothing to do with Roberta's headaches, but her neurosurgeon convinced her to undergo surgery. (She was told that surgery might relieve her headaches but had to be done regardless because of the risk that the malformation could rupture and bleed. In reality, the lifetime risk of that was far less than the risk of surgery.) Fortunately, she made it through surgery safely. Not surprisingly, her headaches persisted.

When she came to me, Roberta was on birth-control pills. She hadn't noticed increased headaches when she first began taking the pills, so she didn't relate them to her headaches that developed a year later. But they sure were related: after she stopped birth-control pills, her headaches stopped. If she'd only done that before the MRI scan, she'd have avoided the scan and the unnecessary brain surgery it led to. ◆

the time of the menstrual cycle. Either way, prescribing hormones for headaches often backfires.

Menstrual headaches are natural (though not necessary). The hormonal shifts—especially just before but also during and right after menses, as well as in midcycle around ovulation—are triggers for migraine. (There's no point in checking blood tests of hormones, because this is *normal*.) Migraine may or may not *actually* be triggered at these times, depending on the levels of other triggers in relation to your threshold, but it is *more likely* to be triggered at these times. (Just a thought: When the symptoms of so-called "premenstrual syndrome" are mainly headache, nausea, dizziness and others common to migraine, doesn't this suggest that in such cases so-called PMS may *be* migraine? Since PMS can otherwise be tough to treat, maybe a migraine-preventive approach—the 1-2-3 Program—is worth trying when these particular symptoms prevail premenstrually.)

It is a mistake to think that headaches regularly related to the menstrual cycle reflect a hormonal "abnormality," and (generally) a greater mistake to try treating headaches with hormonal contraception to "correct" a presumed hormonal imbalance or irregularity.

The use of continuous (noncyclical) hormonal therapy to suppress menses altogether and thereby avoid associated menstrual headaches has a rational foundation but more often acts as fuel, rather than a blanket, on the fire of migraine. The *episodic* triggering effect of menses may be eliminated, but continuous hormonal contraception itself may act as a trigger on a *continuous* basis, thereby raising your baseline trigger level and making headaches and other migraine symptoms worse overall. A good general rule: *If your headaches are not under control, stay away from hormonal contraception.*

Women who use hormonal contraception for reasons beyond birth control—for example, to reduce severe menstrual cramps—should check with their doctor to see if there is an alternative, nonhormonal

Regular Is Better

One situation in which hormones can help control migraine is the use of a short course of progesterone or some other temporary hormonal manipulation to regularize an irregular menstrual pattern. Migraine tends to be more active in response to irregularities of all sorts—including disturbances of your sleep-wake cycle, inconsistent meal patterns and weather changes—and menstrual irregularity is no exception. The downside of a short course of progesterone or some other temporary hormonal manipulation is that it may stimulate headaches temporarily, but this may be a worthwhile price to pay if menstrual irregularity is corrected, promoting better headache control in the long run. ◆

approach. Perhaps menstrual cramps can be controlled with high-dose anti-inflammatory medication. Also, whatever noncontraceptive need for hormonal therapy (such as birth-control pills) there may have been in the past, that need may or may not still exist. Maybe it's worth trying to do without hormones, getting your headaches under control and subsequently attempting to resume hormones—if you want or need to—and seeing what happens. If hormonal contraception *is* used, a low-dose approach is least likely to stimulate headaches. Generally, progestins trigger headaches less than estrogens do.

Occasionally concern arises about hormonal contraception causing stroke in women with active migraine. Some data suggest that, independent of migraine, stroke risk is increased in women taking high-dose birth-control pills, especially combined with cigarette smoking and being over 35 years old. The role of migraine in causing stroke on top of birth-control pill use is unclear, except to say that any effect is relatively small. It is also uncertain, at least in my mind, whether women with especially frequent or severe symptoms of migraine, including neurological symptoms, are necessarily at higher risk of stroke associated with birth-control pills, compared with women with lesser symptoms.

Which Hormones Are Best?

When HRT is used, increased headaches are least likely to occur with the lowest possible dosage of a pure synthetic estrogen, ethinyl estradiol. This is available either as a skin patch (Estraderm, Climara) or orally (Estrace). The skin patch may be better, in that it provides smoother estrogen levels.

From a headache perspective, it's best to take estrogen on a continuous, steady-state basis—rather than cyclically—which is used in conjunction with low-dose progesterone if you still have your uterus. If vaginal dryness is the problem, conjugated estrogen cream or an estradiol vaginal ring (Estring) or tablet (Vagifem) are simple solutions that aren't absorbed into your bloodstream enough to be much of a migraine trigger.

Conversely, cyclical HRT and the use of oral conjugated estrogens such as Premarin, a mixture of estrogens derived from pregnant mares' urine, are relatively more likely to stimulate headaches. "Herbal" or "natural" hormones and dietary hormonal supplements such as soy isoflavones and black cohosh—if they actually do mimic the action of HRT—may well have the potential to stimulate migraine, too. It is unclear whether new forms of HRT such as raloxifene (Evista), which bind more selectively to certain estrogen receptors, are less likely than standard therapy to trigger headaches. ◆

Would a complete hysterectomy, including removal of the ovaries, be a good idea for menstrual headaches? No, don't even think about it. I've seen this backfire—badly—too many times. What usually happens is that the abrupt withdrawal of hormones from sudden surgical menopause leads to a *rise* in headaches that is further fueled when HRT is added.

Don't mess with Mother Nature.

Hormone Replacement Therapy (HRT)
and Other Hormonal Treatments

IMPENDING OR ACTIVE MENOPAUSE can trigger increased (and sometimes altered) migraine symptoms that may persist for a few weeks to a few years. A rise in headaches may be the first clue that menopause is on its way. The natural tendency is for migraine to subside postmenopause, but adding hormone replacement therapy may have the opposite effect. There may be reasons to consider HRT, both short-term (relief of hot flashes, night sweats, insomnia, vaginal dryness and mood disturbances) and long-term (reduced risks of osteoporosis, possibly heart disease and—even more questionably—Alzheimer's disease). Keep in mind that there are other, nonhormonal means to reduce some of these risks, such as biophosphonates—alendronate (Fosamax) and risendronate (Actonel)—for prevention of osteoporosis.

Aside from increased migraine activity, HRT has other potential risks, including breast and uterine cancer. Ideally, from a headache perspective, you should avoid HRT until your headaches are controlled. Then, if you want or need to, you can try HRT, see what happens and decide if the potential benefits outweigh any headaches and other migraine symptoms that result. Remember that increased headaches secondary to HRT sometimes occur months after initiation.

It's trickier if you're already on HRT and are suffering from headaches. One option is to use a different form of HRT. Or, you could eliminate HRT, at least temporarily, but you may have withdrawal symptoms such as hot flashes, insomnia and depression. Or you may not. If you do, these symptoms may subside on their own after a while.

If HRT is mandatory but results in increased headaches, it's all the more important to follow the migraine-preventive diet to keep your trigger level as low as possible. You can also use preventive medication—Step 3—to raise your threshold for migraine in order to keep it above your heightened trigger level (courtesy of HRT).

Hormonal treatments other than HRT—for that matter, virtually any hormonal change, whether natural or medicinal—can trigger migraine. For instance, fertility drugs (e.g., Clomid) and medications used to suppress endometriosis (e.g., Danacrine or Lupron) often provoke migraine—but overall may do you more good (for their intended purpose) than bad (in terms of headaches), particularly if your need for them isn't permanent.

How about men treated with testosterone? It doesn't seem to be as much of a potential trigger as estrogen, but I've seen my share of male patients for whom testosterone seemed to stir up headaches. Again, the pluses and minuses need to be added up in deciding wheter it's worth the trouble. Women, too, are sometimes faced with the issue of testosterone, if they take a form of HRT combining estrogen and testosterone (Estratest)—usually to enhance libido—yet suffer headaches. In that case, it's probably better to switch to estradiol alone, or better yet to eliminate HRT altogether, at least for the time being.

Stress and Depression as Triggers

STRESS—OR TENSION, anxiety, worry, or whatever you want to call it—is a powerful trigger for migraine. So are depression and virtually all other psychological and emotional disturbances. As one of my headache patients said, "I feel my emotions in my head." Sometimes the relationship between stress and migraine is paradoxical, as when headaches occur not during your most stressful times but with the letdown that occurs *after* stress, as on weekends or at the beginning of a vacation.

To some degree, stress is an unavoidable part of life. My approach to controlling headaches emphasizes elimination of dietary and medication triggers, because this you can do readily and because doing so is effective, even in the face of stress. Remember, you have to choose your battles, and for most people the battles over dietary items and medications are the ones most worth fighting (and most easily won) to gain control of headaches. During times of greater stress, it helps to be even more careful about those triggers that you can more readily avoid.

If instead, or in addition, you choose to address stress as a migraine trigger, you can try to reduce either your exposure to stressors or your response to them. Reducing your exposure to stressors may involve cutting back on work, or not taking courses in the evenings, or otherwise juggling fewer balls. Or, you may need to resolve relationships or avoid situations that give rise to stress. The other approach,

---

"The hot flashes weren't so bad"

BETTY'S STORY

Betty was 73 and knew headaches well, having suffered for decades from a frequent assortment that she categorized as "classic migraines," "cluster migraines" and "sinus." But she'd never before experienced the right-sided weakness that lasted five minutes during an otherwise typical classic episode. She was worked up extensively for causes of stroke, and none was found, making it clear (to me) that this was all migraine.

Betty had been taking hormone replacement in the form of Premarin. I made a series of suggestions for the purpose of migraine control, but when she returned to me in four months, it turned out that she'd only needed to do one thing, which was the first thing she did: she switched from Premarin to estradiol. There had been some hot flashes, but they were "tolerable." Remarkably, she had been completely headache-free, *despite enormous stress related to family health problems. (And, no more stroke-like episodes.)* ◆

reducing your response to stressors, may require an attitude change such as deciding that *you* come first. Using the 1-2-3 Program and thereby controlling your headaches helps to encourage a positive attitude change of this sort.

In my experience, biofeedback, relaxation therapy, hypnosis and similar methods of stress management aren't very effective—or at least aren't sufficient—for most headache sufferers. If the idea is to use some such method on a regular basis to manage stress long-term, few people have the time, dedication or ability to do so. If the method is intended as an *acute* intervention, taking time out during a crisis and using the method to relax—well, for most people, in most stressful situations, that's unrealistic.

As for depression and migraine, the two tend to aggravate each other. Being depressed can trigger headaches, and having headaches can be depressing. There may be a shared, underlying neurotransmitter disturbance causing depression and migraine in some people, such that when this disturbance activates it gives rise to both, together. Depression usually is treatable, and as discussed in the next chapter, certain antidepressant medications can also prevent migraine. But when depression and migraine coexist, be careful: some medications used to treat one can make the other worse.

Other Modifiable Triggers

BEYOND DIETARY MODIFICATION, you can make other lifestyle choices to help control your headaches. Regularity is key: you should sleep, eat and exercise on a regular basis. Get enough sleep each night, seven to eight hours or more, and don't oversleep sporadically, as on weekends.

Skipping meals is a common trigger for migraine. Stay on schedule for three meals a day, no more than six to eight hours apart. Snack in between if you wish—but only on nonrestricted items!

Exercise helps both body and mind, and in both ways helps to control headaches. It's not just that regular exercise is a means of relieving stress and thereby reducing your trigger load. Exercise also enhances endorphin production in the brain and is a natural way to help raise your migraine threshold, which otherwise requires preventive medication (Step 3). Aim for a half-hour or more of aerobic exercise three to four times a week. Even if strenuous exertion is a trigger for your headaches when they are not under control, regular exercise can help you gain control. Try warming up gradually, keep well hydrated and consider taking an anti-inflammatory drug such as ibuprofen (up to 800 mg) or naproxen sodium (up to 660 mg) a half hour to an hour beforehand and again four hours or more later if needed.

What's Next?

THE INITIAL GAME PLAN of preventive treatment is to avoid or eliminate rebound, simultaneously eliminate all potential dietary and medication triggers, and see what happens over the next two months. For a few weeks, you may have increased headaches as a result of eliminating quick-fix medications and caffeine. And it can take time to become adept at following the diet: remembering the restricted items, reading labels, adjusting recipes and asking questions about ingredients in meals at restaurants and at other people's homes.

If after two months you're satisfied with your reduced level of headaches (and other migraine symptoms), great. Satisfaction comes when you achieve the sense that you're in control, rather than your headaches and headache treatment having control over you. In that case, keep doing what you've been doing *for at least two months longer—a total of four months*—to be confident that you can maintain control and to develop an enduring memory of what it feels like to have control. In the future, you may need this prolonged memory of *how good it feels* (to be in control) in order to help maintain your motivation to keep doing the right things or to get back on track if you fall off. If, on the other hand, after two months you aren't satisfied with your level of headache control, that's where the next chapter—Step 3—comes in.

The goal is not to *eliminate* your headaches (and other migraine symptoms); it's to eliminate your headache *problem.* The goal is to reduce your headache frequency, severity and duration to a level where you're reasonably satisfied: a situation that you can live with. For those with chronic daily headache, control means having headache-free days—hopefully most days. Part of headache control is being able to manage, tolerate and function despite headaches that still occur from time to time but are milder, briefer and more responsive to simple acute remedies (such as acetaminophen or ibuprofen) that didn't used to work. (My patients often comment that, once they've controlled their headaches fairly well but have occasional breakthroughs, they're amazed to learn that these drugs can actually be effective!)

Reintroducing Potential Triggers

AFTER MAINTAINING HEADACHE CONTROL for four months or more, you can attempt—if you wish—to add back potential triggers one

On Keeping a Diary

I'm not a big fan of headache diaries. The best way to determine dietary triggers is to first control your headaches by avoiding all potential culprits, then carefully begin reintroducing selected items after at least four months problem-free. Just be on the lookout for one or two days after reintroducing a potential trigger; you might get away with a dietary trigger at certain times but not others, depending on your level of other triggers.

The goal of the 1-2-3 Program is to control your headaches to the point where you no longer have a headache *problem.* It seems to me that keeping a diary *declares* a problem by virtue of documenting one, when the whole point is to be able to *ignore* the relatively few, mild headaches you may still have. ◆

at a time and see what happens. If you add back an item and headaches recur, the message is clear: stay away from it. If you add back an item and maintain headache control: so far, so good.

The best way to add back dietary items is to pick the item you miss the most and dedicate a week to it, consuming it daily. If early in the week headaches recur, you can terminate that trial. Just make sure you learn that lesson. If you wish, you can move on to another item. If headaches don't recur by the end of the week, you can probably tolerate that item, at least in the quantities you've consumed up to that point, and without being exposed to an increase in other triggers on top of it.

The rationale for this approach is twofold. First, it allows for the fact that dietary triggers can act on a delayed basis: up to a day or two after consumption. In other words, a weeklong trial gives sufficient time for headaches to catch up with you—if they're going to—as a result of reintroducing that dietary item. Second, over the course of a week your level of other triggers will vary, so you can see more clearly if you'll be able to tolerate that dietary item not only on good days (when you're not otherwise headache-prone) but also on bad days (when you are, because of impending menses, increased stress, sleep deprivation or falling barometric pressure).

The alternative approach to dietary liberalization is to cheat here and there. Frankly, that's the way most of my patients wind up doing it. If you do cheat, don't forget the reasons I just mentioned as to why you might be fooled into thinking you can get away with something even though it really is a trigger for you—at least when you're already hovering near your threshold.

Maintaining Control

YOU'RE WELCOME TO CONTINUE to follow the entire diet strictly if you don't want to rock the boat, at least for now. You can always try relaxing the diet later. It's up to you to decide if the potential

But No Caffeine!

You can work your way down through the list, reintroducing dietary items, *but don't even think about adding back caffeine.* It isn't worth it. Caffeine is among the most potent dietary triggers and consequently the least likely to be tolerated upon reintroduction, at least long-term. But its temporary constricting effects on blood vessels may mislead you into thinking it's helping your headaches, even as it's causing rebound vasodilation and delayed rebound headaches that you may not associate with caffeine because of the delay. Unlike other dietary triggers that you may be able to tolerate with *occasional* usage, consuming caffeine off and on is *especially* likely to stimulate headaches because of the withdrawal headaches that can follow intermittent caffeine exposure.

To whatever extent you think you need caffeine to boost your energy level, you're ignoring the fatigue that follows each time you withdraw from your last dose. Finally, to those who argue that caffeine adds something to the taste of beverages containing it, I say: *Come on.* If it adds anything, it doesn't add that much—just a little bitterness—and certainly not enough to make it worthwhile to suffer recurrent headaches. ◆

pleasure of being able to reintroduce certain of the restricted dietary items outweighs the risk of having recurrent headaches. You can balance dietary sacrifice against headache control to suit your wants and needs.

Don't be surprised if the diet turns out to be a lesser burden than you ever imagined as it lightens you of your headache load. Many of my patients tell me that for them the diet has become a matter of habit—a way of life—and they just stick with it. Others champ at the bit to cut corners and succeed to varying degrees in doing so.

If after achieving and maintaining headache control for four months or more you wish to reintroduce a medication that is a potential trigger, such as birth-control pills, fine, but don't try to liberalize the diet at the same time. Reintroduce potential triggers—either dietary items or medications—*individually* or else you won't be able to identify the cause if headaches recur.

Suppose that after achieving headache control and reintroducing some triggers without apparent difficulty, months later you begin having increased headaches and become dissatisfied again. You need to reverse direction, returning at least for a while to stricter avoidance of triggers. Just because you were able to reintroduce certain dietary items and still avoid headaches for a while doesn't mean these items aren't contributing to your resurgent headaches.

One of two things has happened in this scenario (see Figure 9, page 107). Maybe you've added back too many of the triggers you avoided initially, as a result of which your total trigger level is again above the threshold. Your quantities of these triggers have gradually risen, or you're now consuming them in closer proximity to each other, instead of being as careful as you were when you first started liberalizing the diet. (Remember, the impact of dietary triggers is dose-related. More is worse.) Or, some other trigger, such as increased stress or a hormonal change, has been added to the stack. Whichever is the case, you can reduce your level of triggers by more carefully eliminating the avoidable ones—certain dietary items and medications—that you've reintroduced and thereby restore headache control.

Trigger avoidance can be fine-tuned from day to day. When you wake up feeling a bit heavy-headed or cloudy, you'd be wise to avoid dietary indiscretion that day. Don't push your luck when you're feeling kind of unlucky.

You may find that you can get away with dietary triggers at certain times of the day but not at others. Alcohol, for instance, may be

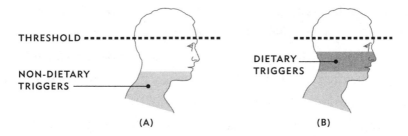

FIGURE 9: RECURRING HEADACHES. *Eliminating dietary triggers from the total trigger load keeps the level below the threshold (A). Reintroducing some dietary triggers raises the level only slightly (B) and migraine remains under control.*

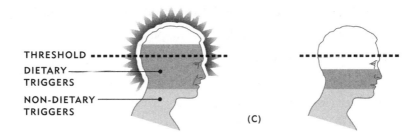

When too many dietary triggers are reintroduced, migraine symptoms are no longer controlled; however, when these triggers are reduced, symptoms are once again under control.

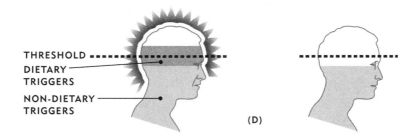

Or, as the result of a rise in some other, nondietary trigger, the total trigger level exceeds the threshold and symptoms recur. Again, by eliminating dietary triggers, symptoms are controlled.

tolerable in the evening but not during the day, especially outside on a sunny, hot summer afternoon. There may be predictable times when you're more prone to headaches because of recurring, unavoidable triggers—as before menstrual periods, or when storms approach, or when traveling by air—and at those times you will do well to take more care in staying away from the avoidable triggers. (On the other hand, if you vacation in France, Italy or some other place far removed from the pressures of your workaday world, you may be so carefree that you can indulge indiscriminately in red wine, cheese, fresh bread and chocolate without getting a headache!)

Over the long haul, you can adjust your degree of trigger avoidance to meet your need for headache control. It's a matter of balancing the burden of headaches against the burden of trigger avoidance. You can find the most comfortable balance for you. In the next chapter, you'll learn how preventive medication can further reduce your headaches, your need for trigger avoidance, or both.

CHAPTER FIVE

Step 3: Raising Your Threshold

You may be able to gain control of your headaches and other migraine symptoms by taking Steps 1 and 2, that is, simply by avoiding rebound and reducing your trigger level below your threshold. Or, despite the first two steps, you may not achieve satisfaction. In that case, Step 3—raising your threshold—comes next. If you've tried regular aerobic exercise as a threshold-elevating measure but still aren't satisfied, it's time to consider migraine-preventive medication.

Remember, the goal is not to eliminate your headaches. The goal is to eliminate your headache *problem*: when the headaches are too frequent, too severe or too long-lasting. They may be a problem for you because they persist in the background, day after day, or they may incapacitate you too often, or both. They're no longer a problem when you feel that you—and not your headaches—are in control.

Do You Need Step 3?

AT WHAT POINT ARE HEADACHES so frequent, so severe or so long-lasting —despite Steps 1 and 2—that preventive medication is justified? That's up to you to judge; it varies from person to person. Imagine being on a seesaw, with you on one end and your headaches on the other. When your headaches are a heavy burden, you're left dangling helplessly in the air. If Steps 1 and 2 lighten your headache load enough, and you've grown strong enough, you'll feel your feet firmly on the ground. Okay, sometimes maybe only your toes are touching, but still you know you're basically in control. Even an occasional bounce up in the air isn't a big deal, because you've learned that you'll be back on the ground soon enough. You know where your tipping point is, and how to get back on the right side of it.

If you find yourself on the right end of the headache seesaw after Steps 1 and 2, continue doing what you've been doing for at least another two months. At that point, you may be able to reintroduce an infrequent quick fix or certain potential triggers. But if you still feel helpless, at the mercy of your headaches, it's time to move on to Step 3: an effective preventive medication taken daily. Maybe you don't want to take such a medication every day, but it sure makes more sense than suffering from relentless headaches and gobbling counterproductive quick fixes by the fistful.

Why wait until this point to add preventive medication? That is, why not add it at the start? First, because you might never need it, and if you find yourself doing well enough (courtesy of Steps 1 and 2) but happen to be on preventive medication already, you might give *it* the credit and be reluctant to give it up . . . even though you don't need it. Second, you might blame the potentially unpleasant symptoms of withdrawal from quick fixes and dietary caffeine on any preventive medication that you happen to have started around the same time and develop such a bad taste for it that you'll never try it again, even though it was an innocent bystander and would have been well tolerated and worked great once the dust settled. And third, preventive medication won't work well *until* the dust has settled, which is where we are now.

But wait. Before you move on to Step 3, remember that you must *continue* Steps 1 and 2. They may not have been *sufficient* to control your headaches, but they are nonetheless *necessary* in order for Step 3 to be effective. You mustn't backstep on the path to headache control.

The Principles of Preventive Medication

WITH ONE MINOR EXCEPTION, no medication used for migraine prevention was designed for this purpose. The discovery that certain medications can prevent migraine came from incidental observations of decreased headaches among people taking them for other purposes.

Exactly how these medications work to prevent migraine is unclear, but in effect they raise the threshold for migraine by blocking one or more neurotransmitters in their pathway. This makes the mechanism harder to trigger, or less fully activated even if it *is* triggered (see Figure 10, page 115). You can think of these medications as threshold elevators.

The effectiveness of any preventive medication depends on maintaining an adequate level in your system, which means you have to take it daily. As a general rule, preventive medications don't work well after the fact; that is, they help to avoid the triggering of migraine but are less effective when taken after the mechanism has been set into motion.

Here are the guidelines for proper use of preventive medication. See Table 9 (page 112–13) for a medication that has a good chance of working. Try one at a time. Start with a low dosage to avoid initial

Migraine-Preventive Medication

MEDICATION	INITIAL DOSAGE	MAXIMAL DOSAGE or BLOOD LEVEL
TRICYCLIC ANTIDEPRESSANTS Nortriptyline or amitriptyline	10 or 25 mg at bedtime	100 to 200 mg at bedtime or level greater than 200 to 250 ng/ml
CALCIUM CHANNEL BLOCKERS Verapamil or diltiazem	120 mg once or twice daily	240 to 360 mg twice daily
DIVALPROEX	125 to 250 mg at bedtime or ER (extended release) 500 mg at bedtime	1,000 mg twice daily or level greater than 200 mcg/ml

BETA BLOCKERS
    Nadolol
    Propanolol
	20 to 40 mg daily
	40 to 80 mg daily
		80 mg twice daily
		160 mg twice daily

CYPROHEPTADINE	2 to 4 mg at bedtime	8 mg three times daily

NONSTEROIDAL ANTI-INFLAMMATORY DRUGS
    Ibuprofen
    Naproxen
    Celecoxib
    Rofecoxib
	400 mg three times daily
	220 mg twice daily
	100 mg daily
	25 mg daily
		800 mg four times daily
		660 mg three times daily
		200 mg twice daily
		50 mg daily

CORTICOSTEROIDS Prednisone	20 to 80 mg daily, then taper	—
METHYSERGIDE	2 mg twice daily	4 mg three times daily

VIRTUES	VICES
Also good for insomnia, depression, anxiety	Possible dry mouth, sedation, constipation, increased appetite
Well tolerated; also treats high blood pressure	Possible constipation
Also good for seizures, manic-depressive illness	Possible nausea, tremor, hair loss, sedation, increased appetite
Also treat high blood pressure and certain heart conditions	Possible fatigue, insomnia, depression; may be a problem with asthma or diabetes
Can function as antihistamine for allergies	Possible sedation, increased appetite
Can be used *intermittently* for prevention, as around menses, or before exertion	Not usually highly effective; possible stomach irritation
Useful for brief treatment of "crises"	*Many* side effects, especially if used long-term
Rarely, will work when all else fails	Serious side effects in small percentage of users

Table 9

Why "Failed" Headache Patients Have Failed

You now understand that you must establish a proper setting in order for any preventive medication (Step 3) to be most effective. This means you must first avoid or eliminate rebound (Step 1) and reduce your exposure to avoidable triggers as much as possible (Step 2).

Before coming to me, most of my new patients failed multiple trials of preventive medications because they didn't take the first two steps. As with most things in life that are to succeed, first things must come first. Rebound was not avoided, or dietary and medication triggers were not restricted carefully enough. Predictably, their preventive medication treatment failed again and again, and they came to me labeled as "failed" headache patients—with the obvious implication that *they* were failures.

By the time I see them, these patients usually have a "been everywhere, done everything" attitude about their headache treatment and generally feel on the brink of hopelessness. But they're *not* hopeless, and they're not failures. These individuals *do* respond to preventive treatment, *but it must start with the basics—* Steps 1 and 2. In fact, with the proper foundation of preventive treatment, Step 3 is not even necessary for many or even most chronic headache sufferers. And it may not be for you. Either way, you must start with the basics. ◆

---

side effects. Keep increasing the dosage slowly but steadily over a period of two months until you either achieve satisfactory headache control or hit the dosage ceiling. The therapeutic benefit of these medications is dose-related: the higher the dosage, the higher your threshold rises. Sometimes just a small increment in dosage is all it takes to raise your threshold above your trigger level and thereby control your headaches.

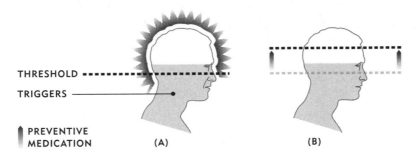

THRESHOLD

TRIGGERS

PREVENTIVE
MEDICATION   (A)   (B)

FIGURE 10: RAISING THE THRESHOLD. *Without preventive medication, triggers stack up and symptoms occur (A). Preventive medication raises the threshold (B) so that symptoms are now controlled.*

The Common Mistakes

DOCTORS OFTEN MAKE the same mistakes in prescribing preventive medication: too much too soon, too little or too many. It's a mistake to push up the dosage too rapidly; "intolerable side effects" often turn out to be tolerable (or nonexistent) if higher dosages are reached more gradually. On the other hand, it's a mistake to let preventive medication trials drag on forever at ineffectively low dosages. If you add or change multiple medications at once, it's difficult to determine why you're then better, or worse, or (in different ways) both; plus, their side effects often multiply.

There are two ways to determine your dosage ceiling: (1) by intolerable side effects that cannot be circumvented by, for example, lowering the dosage and raising it again more gradually, or (2) by maximal allowable dosage. For some medications, maximal allowable dosage is a certain number of milligrams per day, and for others it's determined by measuring blood levels or checking an electrocardiogram (EKG) to look for any adverse effect on the electrical activity of the heart. Make sure you go *all the way up to the ceiling* before you conclude that a given medication isn't effective.

Don't look for trouble when it comes to side effects. If you convince yourself before starting that a medication will cause side effects, you'll probably never take it long enough or at high enough dosage to benefit. If you keep this up, you'll talk yourself into intolerance of one medication after another, even at very low dosages. Don't script yourself into this self-fulfilling prophecy. And be sure to ask yourself what's wrong with this picture if you supposedly can't tolerate *any* preventive medication but have *no* problem with frequent use of potent quick fixes.

Used properly, each of the preventive medications in Table 9 (pages 112–13) has a two-thirds or better likelihood of helping you. Used improperly, as is too often the case, these drugs have a much lower success rate. If one drug within a group of similar drugs hasn't worked under proper conditions, its cousins probably won't, either. *Be patient.* If you keep trying different types of preventive medication *properly,* you can find one that will work for you.

Dealing with Potential Side Effects

TAKING ANY PREVENTIVE MEDICATION means you *may* have to deal with nuisance side effects. As a rule, the higher the dosage, the greater the likelihood of side effects. But there are exceptions; sometimes you gain better headache control with only minimally (if at all) increased side effects by going up with the dosage. You can fine-tune the dosage, balancing benefit against side effects.

Many side effects will diminish if you give yourself a chance to adjust. This may be contrary to your intuition. You might think: *If my mouth is so dry (or I'm so sedated, or whatever) this soon after starting the medication, I bet it'll get even worse if I keep taking it!*

Actually, it's the other way around. Side effects tend to subside over time. Impatience with initial side effects can undermine trials of preventive medications that would have worked well in the long run—if there had been a long run. Each time the dosage is increased, the same adjustment may need to take place; and each time you should be patient. In the event that an initial nuisance side effect is unbearable, the dosage can be reduced temporarily and then increased again after a while, but more gently. Unless you have certain underlying medical problems, which your doctor would know about, serious complications from preventive medications are rare.

"I was almost never without a headache"

JEAN'S STORY

*A*fter years of ineffective allergy shots and other misguided treatments, Jean came to me with headaches that were especially bad around her periods ("head-hangers," she called them), but she had to admit that she also had at least a "low-grade" headache nearly every day.

Jean has done "really great" overall and even "perfectly," with no headaches for several months in a row, at times. How? She's stayed away from her previous quick fixes (Esgic Plus, Zomig and Maxalt); she's followed the diet "pretty darn carefully"; and she's taken the tricyclic antidepressant nortriptyline for migraine prevention. Jean uses a low dose of 25 mg most of the month and goes up to 50 mg for a week around her periods.

P.S.: On nortriptyline, Jean's "PMS" mood swings have leveled off, and she sleeps much more soundly. Her mouth was dry at first—a price well worth paying for the benefits she's gained—but even that's getting better now. ◆

What About Pregnancy and Breast-Feeding?

The most common reason for not being a candidate for preventive medication is pregnancy, either actual or potential. Ideally, you should not take preventive medication if you're attempting to become pregnant and should avoid it, if possible, throughout pregnancy. Fortunately, many chronic headache sufferers find a respite in pregnancy; however, headache activity can go either way during pregnancy, and especially in the beginning it may go up. In uncommon, desperate situations where a woman might need a preventive medication during pregnancy, only certain options are reasonable, and this decision should involve both the obstetrician and a headache specialist.

Breast-feeding poses similar but lesser concerns, and the baby's pediatrician needs to advise whether any given preventive medication is acceptable in that setting. Often women don't menstruate until they stop breast-feeding, and they don't have recurrent headaches until they resume menstruation. In this case, breast-feeding itself may help prevent headaches! ◆

Adding and Adjusting Preventive Medication

IF A GIVEN PREVENTIVE MEDICATION is ineffective despite a fair trial lasting two months, with appropriate upward dosage adjustment combined with Step 1 (absence of rebound) and Step 2 (avoidance of all potential dietary and medication triggers), it's time to eliminate it and move on to the next option. On the other hand, if a preventive medication is *somewhat* though not satisfactorily effective after a full, fair trial, you should continue it for the time being and add a second preventive medication to it.

In this scenario, if the addition of a second medication achieves headache control, you and your doctor can then try to reduce or eliminate the first medication, which may no longer be needed. Some people do require two or, rarely, three preventive medications, but additions should be made one at a time, and in the long run subtraction of medication should be considered since not all may be needed long-term.

How long do you need to take preventive medication? The answer is: as long as you need to. You can periodically try to reduce or even eliminate your medication—gradually, one at a time—to see if you can maintain control of your headaches without it. Migraine activity fluctuates as thresholds and trigger levels rise and fall for reasons that may or may not be identifiable, and you may need preventive medication to help control your headaches this month or this year, but not next.

But there is another factor to consider. The more strictly you avoid dietary and medication triggers, the less preventive medication you will require (see Figure 11, page 120). Conversely, the less carefully you stay away from avoidable triggers, the more preventive medication you will require to achieve control of headaches and other migraine symptoms. You can balance the extent to which you avoid triggers, the amount of preventive medication you take and your level of headache control to best suit your needs and desires. But I recommend that you focus *primarily* on trigger avoidance—and secondarily rely on preventive medication—in order to minimize your medication exposure. (And don't forget the value of regular exercise as both a trigger reducer and a threshold elevator.)

If you don't want to risk attempting to reduce (or eliminate) preventive medication, or if you've tried and have suffered renewed headaches as a consequence, don't fret. These medications are generally safe even in the long run. You can also *increase* the dosage of preventive medication temporarily if needed—for example, around menstrual periods, or intermittently during stressful times, or just for a few days if you have a persistent, bad headache for whatever reason. The idea is to boost your threshold in order to reestablish it above a temporarily

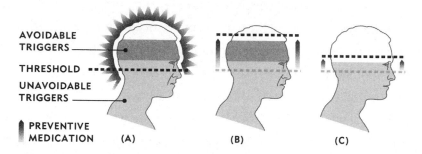

FIGURE 11: ELIMINATING AVOIDABLE TRIGGERS. *Before medication, a heavy load of both unavoidable and avoidable triggers pushes the overall level far above the threshold (A). A high dosage of preventive medication is needed to raise the threshold high enough to control symptoms (B). When avoidable triggers are eliminated, the threshold doesn't need to be so high and therefore less preventive medication is required (C).*

elevated trigger level. Increasing the dosage temporarily may increase some nuisance side effects, but that may be a worthwhile price to pay, at least short-term, for better headache control at such times.

Choosing a Preventive Medication

WHICH PREVENTIVE MEDICATION might be best for you? It depends on your coexisting conditions and potential vulnerability to certain side effects, as well as the outcome of any prior preventive medication trials. Look at prior trials with a critical eye on their inadequacies, rather than thinking that you've exhausted each option. More often than not, it's worth trying "failed" medications again—this time the right way.

In prior trials you may have had intolerable side effects because a medication was started at excessive dosage, whereas from a lower, tolerable initial dosage you could build gradually and successfully. The maximal dosage you took may not have been enough; perhaps you could benefit from higher dosage. Too many drugs at once may have clouded the picture by magnifying side effects or by interfering with each other, especially if quick fixes caused rebound and blocked your ability to respond to preventive medication. You may have paid inadequate attention to avoiding dietary triggers or birth-control pills or other medication triggers. The bottom line is: failed preventive medication trials are likely to have been inadequate, and often the wisest course is to start from scratch, considering *all* the potential options rather than ruling out those that have *unfairly* failed in the past.

The preventive medication that is best for you is not determined by the details of your migraine problem. Preventive medications are roughly interchangeable in their threshold-elevating effect, regardless of your particular migraine symptoms. The best choice is determined by consideration of your health status in other respects. The right preventive medication may be a stone that kills two or even three birds. The wrong choice may help control migraine, but at needless expense in some other regard.

Here are some examples of wise choices: a tricyclic antidepressant for migraine if you also suffer from insomnia, depression or anxiety; certain calcium channel blockers or beta blockers for migraine if you also have high blood pressure or heart disease; and divalproex for migraine if you're also troubled by seizures or psychiatric problems such as manic-depressive illness. On the other hand, beta blockers, while effective for migraine, are likely to make you feel worse if you're fatigued or depressed or have trouble sleeping to begin with. Or certain medications for depression can stimulate migraine and may be counterproductive when the two problems coexist.

With few exceptions—namely, divalproex (Depakote), propranolol (Inderal), timolol (Blocadren) and methysergide (Sansert)—migraine-preventive medications are not formally approved by the U.S. Food and Drug Administration for this purpose. Their use in migraine prevention is considered "off label" but is nonetheless safe and standard care. This may be an issue for the prescribing doctor, but needn't concern you.

Generic versions of preventive medications tend to be cheaper and are usually adequate, but once in a while the brand-name variety seems to work better for certain individuals, presumably because the dosage delivery is more reliable.

Tricyclics and Other Antidepressants

AMITRIPTYLINE (ELAVIL), imipramine (Tofranil) and desipramine (Norpramin) all belong to this group, but I favor nortriptyline (Pamelor) because it is less likely to cause nuisance side effects. Although the effect of tricyclics in preventing migraine is independent of treating depression, the common coincidence of migraine and depression makes tricyclics an especially good fit in such cases. But you don't have to be depressed to benefit from these medications; they work well on migraine alone.

Most people who take tricyclics experience dry mouth due to decreased salivation. This is usually tolerable but can be further managed by sipping liquids, chewing gum or sucking on lozenges. Decreased salivation can increase your risk of cavities, so take good care of your teeth and use sugarless lozenges or gum (preferably without aspartame, a potential migraine trigger). Synthetic saliva spray is also available.

Tricyclics can cause constipation, which you can alleviate by increasing your dietary fiber and fluid intake and exercising more. If needed, you can use a fiber supplement or stool softener. Tricyclics also sometimes stimulate appetite, which occasionally leads to weight gain, especially if you overeat and don't exercise regularly.

The primary dose-limiting side effect of tricyclics is sedation (which may be a plus if you're an insomniac). For this reason tricyclics are usually taken once a day at bedtime, but if you're still left feeling groggy in the morning, try taking it earlier in the evening or at dinnertime. Remember, side effects tend to diminish over time, so whatever sedation you experience when you initiate or escalate a tricyclic is likely to subside within a few days or weeks. If it's too much to handle, you can cut back on the dosage and raise it more slowly later.

A few individuals find tricyclics stimulating rather than sedating and become restless after taking the medication near bedtime, so they do better taking it in the morning. The dosage can be split between morning and evening, if you prefer. Nortriptyline is available in 10, 25, 50 and 75 mg capsules, and combinations of 10 and 25 mg capsules allow for dosage increments of as little as 5 mg. For example, three 10 mg capsules equals 30 mg, and one 10 mg plus one 25 mg capsule adds up to 35 mg. Nortriptyline in liquid form—2 mg per 1 ml—permits even finer tuning.

There's a tendency for doctors to be overly preoccupied with blood levels of tricyclic antidepressants, and sometimes, when the level is relatively high, the test result imposes an artificially (and unfortunately) low ceiling on the dosage in patients who seem to be tolerating the medication just fine but might benefit from even higher dosage. I suggest monitoring with EKGs (rather than blood levels) when the dosage is relatively high but might go even higher, because EKGs better reflect any potential disturbance of electrical activity of the heart, which is the major concern about high-dose tricyclic antidepressant toxicity.

Antidepressants other than tricyclics, including selective serotonin reuptake inhibitors (SSRIs) such as fluoxetine (Prozac), paroxetine (Paxil), sertraline (Zoloft), citalopram (Celexa) and fluvoxamine (Luvox), generally are not effective migraine-preventive medications. While there are exceptions to this rule (people who have fewer headaches when taking an SSRI), SSRIs more often *stimulate* headaches—if they have any effect on headaches at all. The same is true of buproprion (Wellbutrin) and venlafaxine (Effexor). If you have both depression and headaches and are taking one of these drugs, you might benefit—at least in terms of headaches—from adding or substituting a tricyclic.

Tranks? No, Thanks!

Tranquilizers, benzo-
diazepines such
as Xanax, Ativan
and Valium in particular,
are prescribed all too
often for all kinds of reasons, including head-
aches. Sure, they might
make you feel better
temporarily. And if your
stress level is sky-high,
you may even benefit in
terms of reduced head-
aches. But these habit-
forming drugs are
usually not good long-
term solutions. I've seen
too many patients suffer-
ing from headaches *and*
depression who felt better
at first on these drugs
but after a while were
sucked into a whirlpool
of declining mood and
function . . . not to mention never-ending head-
aches. When properly
treated, as with a tricyclic
antidepressant for both
migraine and depres-
sion, they can overcome
their headaches *and*
their dependence on
tranquilizers. ◆

Monoamine oxidase inhibitors (MAOIs), including phenelzine (Nardil) and tranylcypromine (Parnate), are antidepressants that are not used very often, largely because of concerns about dangerous elevations of blood pressure if they're combined with certain foods (that contain tyramine) or certain other medications (such as adrenaline-like drugs). But they can be effective for not only depression but also, in some individuals, migraine prevention (though I have prescribed them only rarely). A convenient plus is that the dietary restrictions necessary while taking an MAOI turn out to overlap with the migraine-preventive diet, which also excludes tyramine-containing items.

Calcium Channel Blockers

CALCIUM CHANNEL BLOCKERS are used to treat high blood pressure and certain forms of heart disease as well as for migraine prevention. Among this group, verapamil (Calan, Isoptin, Veralan and Covera-HS) and diltiazem (Cardizem and Tiazac) are the two drugs of choice for migraine; the others don't work well. Verapamil or diltiazem is an especially good choice if you have both migraine and high blood pressure, but either one works just fine for migraine alone.

Verapamil—my particular preference among calcium channel blockers, I suppose mainly just because I've prescribed it more often—and diltiazem are usually well tolerated and therefore are good options if you're especially sensitive to medication side effects such as sedation or increased appetite. Constipation is the most common nuisance side effect and can be managed as with tricyclics. (Diltiazem tends to be less constipating than verapamil.) Occasionally these drugs cause swelling of the feet (if this happens to you, reduce your salt intake and prop up your feet), or they may make you more aware of your heartbeat, which is curious but not problematic.

A common error in adjusting the dosage of verapamil and diltiazem (as well as beta blockers) is to worry too much about lower blood pressure or slower pulse rate. Even though these medications are used

---

"I never thought one pill would be the answer to my prayers"

JERMAINE'S STORY

Jermaine's problem turned out to be so simple to control, it was all the more a shame that he had suffered for so long through endless, fruitless efforts to treat his "tension headaches" with physical therapy, biofeedback, chiropractic manipulation, acupuncture, injections, massage and counseling.

I wrote a letter to Jermaine's primary doctor suggesting that his blood pressure medicine be switched to verapamil, which would not only treat his high blood pressure but also prevent migraine— the true cause of his chronic headaches. The medicine was switched, Jermaine's headaches subsided and he was "extremely satisfied." Two years later he still is, with headaches "once in a blue moon," usually when he cheats too much on the diet. ◆

to treat *high* blood pressure, they don't as a rule, have much effect on blood pressure that is *normal* or *low* to start. Even if your blood pressure or pulse drops with treatment, it generally doesn't matter unless you develop intolerable lightheadedness when you stand up quickly. *Don't look for trouble* by routinely checking your blood pressure and pulse, worrying that they might be too low because you're taking one of these medications, unless you have good reason to believe that you're feeling poorly as a result.

Divalproex

INITIALLY, DIVALPROEX (DEPAKOTE) was marketed for control of seizures, but it is now also formally approved by the FDA for prevention of migraine and treatment of manic-depressive illness. It works well but may cause more nuisance side effects than tricyclic antidepressants and calcium channel blockers, so for me it is a second- rather than a first-line option. Having said that, divalproex may be the best choice for you. This is especially true if it would also be appropriate for coexisting seizures or manic-depressive illness, but it may also be the best choice for you simply because it works effectively to control migraine and is well tolerated.

Potential nuisance side effects of divalproex include nausea, sedation, weight gain (due at least partly to increased appetite), hand tremor, and change in hair texture leading to hair breakage and loss. These side effects are dose-related and are reversible if the medication is stopped. Taking a multivitamin with zinc and selenium may help to avoid the potential hair changes. The manufacturer touts an extended-release form of divalproex as being less likely to cause side effects.

Liver damage in people taking divalproex for migraine is extremely unlikely, but prudence dictates periodic blood tests at the start. Hormonal disturbances have been reported, leading to problems with menstruation and fertility. You shouldn't become pregnant on divalproex (Depakote ER), because it can cause fetal spinal malformations. This list of side effects

Should You Try Neurontin or Topamax or . . . ?

A bunch of relatively new antiseizure medications, such as gabapentin (Neurontin), topiramate (Topamax), lamotrigine (Lamictal), levetiracetam (Keppra) and tiagabine (Gabitril), have spread like wildfire and are now used for all sorts of purposes beyond seizure control—including migraine prevention. They have their proponents, and there are limited studies suggesting benefit, but I haven't been impressed by the response of patients who have tried these drugs before coming to see me.

Maybe these patients didn't receive fair trials because of rebound or inadequate trigger avoidance, and maybe I'm therefore missing the boat. If so, eventually one of these medications, if actually effective, will stand out from the crowd of other supposed migraine-preventive agents that don't really work. (Topamax, in particular, would be a welcome addition to the toolbox because it sometimes leads to weight loss, unlike several of the established preventive medications that occasionally are associated with weight gain.)

The practice of medicine is not immune to fads. In fact, time and again new medications enjoy meteoric rises in popularity, only to wear out their welcome as their initial promise turns out to have been hype. When it comes to medications, newer isn't always better; older, tried and true often is. ◆

ought not scare you away from a potential trial of divalproex; it's a valuable option among preventive medications, and most people tolerate it well.

Beta Blockers

USED TO TREAT high blood pressure and some forms of heart disease, beta blockers are mainstays for migraine prevention but can aggravate fatigue, sluggishness, insomnia and depression, and may be contra-indicated in the face of asthma, diabetes and certain heart conditions. Among the beta blockers, I favor nadolol (Corgard), but propranolol (Inderal), timolol (Blocadren) and metoprolol (Lopressor) are potentially effective. Atenolol (Tenormin) doesn't seem to work as well for migraine sufferers.

Cyproheptadine

CYPROHEPTADINE (PERIACTIN) is an antihistamine (used to relieve problems such as itching) that also affects serotonin receptors and thereby can block migraine. Sedation and increased appetite are potential side effects. Every few months, when a patient who failed trials of other preventive medications has excellent response to (and tolerance of) cyproheptadine, I am reminded what a useful drug it can be for migraine prevention.

Nonsteroidal Anti-Inflammatory Drugs

NONSTEROIDAL ANTI-INFLAMMATORY DRUGS (NSAIDs), including ibuprofen, naproxen and many others, can be used not only for acute headache relief—without risk of rebound—but also for headache prevention. These drugs are especially suitable for menstruation-related headaches, for which an NSAID can be taken on a scheduled basis for several days or more around menses and then discontinued until the next go-round.

NSAIDs can also be used intermittently for prevention of exertional headaches, particularly those that occur with specific activities such as sexual intercourse, weight lifting or jogging. If you're predisposed to exertional headaches, you might benefit from taking an NSAID shortly before exertion and repeating it shortly after. Potential side effects of NSAIDs include stomach irritation (often avoided by taking the medication with food) and gastrointestinal bleeding. Celecoxib (Celebrex) and rofecoxib (Vioxx), two newer, more selective

NSAIDs, are less irritating to the stomach. Chronic usage of NSAIDs can lead to kidney problems, especially in some people who are already predisposed by high blood pressure or diabetes.

Corticosteroids

PREDNISONE AND OTHER CORTICOSTEROIDS are powerful anti-inflammatory agents that can be used to treat a wide variety of conditions, including

"I can't tell if I'm depressed because of my headaches, or vice versa"

LISA'S STORY

L isa's situation was delicate. She suffered both from a mood disorder, tending mainly to depression but with a few manic episodes in recent years, and from chronic headaches. At one point she'd gotten heavily into prescription narcotics for headaches. Not surprisingly, her emotional state bottomed out at that time and her headaches escalated from rebound. Fortunately she detoxified, yet her headaches persisted, worsening her mood and thus causing even more headaches.

When she first came to see me, Lisa was taking Inderal (propranolol) for migraine prevention and Prozac for depression. Ironically—and unfortunately—Inderal was aggravating her depression and Prozac was stimulating migraine. Working with her psychiatrist and her primary doctor, we adjusted her medications, eliminating the Inderal and Prozac and adding Depakote (divalproex). Aside from some mild initial weight gain, Lisa has felt remarkably better than she's felt in years, with stable moods and relatively few headaches. ◆

Botox Shots?

Botox is botulinum toxin, a powerful muscle-paralyzing agent produced by bacteria that could kill you if you ate a jarful of something contaminated by it. Purified and injected, it has found an ever-growing number of medical uses ranging from treating disabling neurological conditions to smoothing wrinkles.

In the course of certain of these uses, such as injections around the head for cosmetic purposes, Botox has seemed to help some people's headaches, and a few small studies have suggested that this effect is for real. But others have not, and it's hard to imagine how it works. Remember, headaches do *not* arise from excessive muscle contraction. Moreover, I've seen quite a few patients who tried Botox, yet I can't think of one who was satisfied with the result. ◆

migraine. They have many potential side effects, but short courses may be appropriate for temporary migraine control in selected circumstances, such as a prolonged "crisis" that won't otherwise respond, or during withdrawal from rebound.

Methysergide

METHYSERGIDE (SANSERT) is indicated exclusively for migraine prevention but isn't used much because of concern about potentially serious complications of fibrosis (scarring) affecting the kidneys, heart or lungs, even though these complications are uncommon. After six months of continuous usage, a one-month drug holiday is advised to help avoid any such problem. Methysergide also has other, less serious potential side effects. But it can be effective, and in a small number of patients it's a reasonable last resort.

What Else Should You Know?

NOW THAT YOU UNDERSTAND what migraine is, and know each of the three steps you can take to control your headaches and the other symptoms it generates, is that the end of the story? Not by a long shot. Next we need to look more carefully at the pervasive myths that, unless exposed, will continue to cloud your recognition of migraine. As I

Vitamins, Minerals and Herbs?

Taking a high-potency multivitamin daily is a good idea, not to prevent headaches but to avoid nutritional complications of dietary modification. There are those who tout high-dose riboflavin—vitamin B$_2$ 400 mg daily—to prevent migraine. Some of my patients have tried it; most haven't been impressed, and neither have I. Magnesium (400 mg once or twice daily), feverfew, butterbur extract, ginger and topical peppermint oil (applied to the forehead or temples) are of dubious benefit, but I don't object to them . . . or to St. John's wort, if you choose to use it for depression. But stay away from other herbs: they can't be trusted *not* to contain potential migraine triggers.

Don't believe that any drug—*including* herbs, which *are* drugs—can work without risk of side effects. Any drug that can help *must be able to harm*. Whether pharmaceutical or herbal, drugs act chemically, and chemical action is not magical. Depending on many factors, some that are known and most that aren't, the chemical action of any drug, including an herb, can lead to an adverse reaction.

Be especially careful of herbal remedies touted to boost energy, promote weight loss or treat "sinus" problems. These may contain caffeine, ephedra, decongestants or other, similar agents that may relieve headaches temporarily by constricting blood vessels but thereby can cause rebound. Other herbal remedies and nutritional "supplements" may include other hidden migraine triggers—such as MSG—and are best avoided. ◆

reveal these myths—and the myriad misdiagnoses they propagate—I'm sure that many will sound familiar to you and touch close to home. You'll realize just how *common* are the problems that stem from migraine (even though they might be called something else) and that you, your family and your friends can *control* these problems using the 1-2-3 Program.

MIGRAINE MYTHS AND

MISDIAGNOSES

CHAPTER SIX

"Tension" and "Sinus" Headaches

From the womb of conventional wisdom, headache myths give birth to headache misdiagnoses. Conventional wisdom would have you believe that there are innumerable different types of headaches with distinctive characteristics and separate mechanisms. In reality, the mechanism of migraine generates virtually all headaches (the main exception being cluster headache, which is related to migraine but stands apart, as explained in Chapter Ten). Still, most headaches are misdiagnosed because they don't conform to the traditional definition of migraine. And misdiagnosis begets mistreatment, which begets needless suffering and frustration.

According to conventional wisdom, the three most prevalent types of headaches are tension headache, sinus headache and migraine. Two of the three types—tension and sinus—are mythical.

Tension headache, also known as stress or muscle-contraction headache, is supposedly characterized by mild-to-moderate, diffuse, nonspecific pain, unassociated with nausea, photophobia and the other features that supposedly define "migraine." Allegedly, tension headache arises from excessive muscle contraction around the head and neck, caused by pent-up emotional disturbances such as tension, stress, anxiety, worry or depression. Sinus headache, the next most prevalent diagnosis, is a label applied to congestion, pressure and pain behind the face (or elsewhere around the head), presumed to arise from a sinus allergy, infection or structural abnormality—or some combination thereof.

Let's take a closer look at these headache myths and the misdiagnoses they spawn.

The Myth of Tension Headache

I WAS TAUGHT—as most doctors were taught, and still believe—that tension headache accounts for the vast majority of chronic headaches. Admittedly, this concept has a certain appeal. When you have a mild-to-moderate headache, your neck may also feel stiff and sore, with a "muscular" quality to the discomfort. The frequent association between stress and an achy head or a "knot" in your neck supports the notion that "tensing up" is the cause. When an activity that you perform in a certain posture leads to a headache, you naturally suspect that the headache has some musculoskeletal basis.

The idea that this type of headache arises from muscular tension or strain is popularly assumed—but simply false. Electrical studies measuring muscle contraction around the head and neck during this type of headache do *not* demonstrate excessive or abnormal activity. Tense muscles are *not* the source of your head and neck pain.

This has long been known by headache specialists, but unfortunately not only most headache sufferers but also most doctors haven't gotten the word and consequently the (mis)diagnosis of tension headache persists. Even failure of treatment doesn't raise questions. Failure is

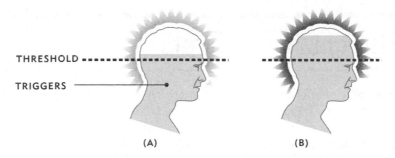

THRESHOLD

TRIGGERS

(A)   (B)

FIGURE 12: THE SPECTRUM OF MIGRAINE. *A trigger load just above the threshold produces mild symptoms—a "tension headache"— as the mechanism is barely activated (A). Continuing to climb (B), the higher trigger level "revs up" the mechanism until "a migraine" occurs.*

half expected anyway, and it can be explained and managed by blaming you, the patient, who then bear the guilt. Meanwhile, your headaches go on and on, unrelieved and unremitting, yet the myth survives.

When Migraine Idles

MIGRAINE, NOT MUSCLE CONTRACTION, is what causes headaches ascribed to tension. These mild-to-moderate, nonspecific headaches stem from low-level activation of the mechanism of migraine, resulting in low-grade swelling and inflammation of blood vessels around your head. Tension and stress *are* potent headache triggers, but they act in concert with other triggers—dietary items, hormones, barometric pressure changes and so on—to turn on migraine. Tension and stress do not cause headaches by causing muscle contraction.

Think of the way a car engine works. When you turn the key in the ignition, the engine starts. If you don't put your foot on the gas pedal, the engine just idles. In the case of migraine, the key in the ignition is turned—and the engine starts—when your triggers rise above your threshold for activation (see Figure 12, above). At this point the

Recognizing the Truth

Shortly after I finished my training, I began advising preventive treatment for patients who came to me complaining of severe headaches that I recognized as migraine, and repeatedly they reported control of these headaches *as well as* relief of their daily "tension" headache.

It took awhile, but eventually I learned that treatment to prevent migraine—specific treatment that would *not* alleviate headache if it were due to muscle contraction—can control not only headaches generally recognized as migraine but also those mislabeled as tension-type. Since both varieties of headaches respond to migraine-preventive treatment, the underlying mechanism of both must be migraine.

Often these patients hadn't even bothered to mention daily headache in the first place. They regarded it as a fact of life. It's understandable. Even something as unpleasant as daily headache can become so embedded in your life that it no longer stands out. If you feel guilty about your headaches, believing that some personal shortcoming is the cause, they become even more difficult to face, so you more readily deny them. Or if you learn early on that your complaints will be greeted with strange looks or snide remarks, you figure it's better to keep quiet.

Here's a helpful question that often leads to full disclosure: How many times a week do you take *any* kind of medication for *any* kind of discomfort around your head, face or neck? Even people who at first complain of headaches only a few times per month often acknowledge that they take *some* kind of medication much more often than that.

Herein lies rich but bitter irony. On the one hand, most chronic headache sufferers *downplay* the full extent of their headaches. On the other hand, many doctors regard headache patients as habitual complainers, because they persistently complain of headaches despite the doctors' best efforts "by the book." What these doctors don't understand is that *the book is wrong*, and by following it *they* are largely responsible for the persistent complaints of their patients. ◆

mechanism is barely activated, or idling, and your symptoms are mild: a "tension headache." If you press your foot down on the gas pedal, or if your triggers climb higher above your threshold, the engine revs up and the mechanism becomes more fully activated. You therefore experience increased headache, nausea, photophobia . . . "a migraine."

Reuniting the Spectrum of Migraine

DESPITE THE MISGUIDED diagnostic efforts of conventional wisdom to carve up the spectrum of migraine into many separate little pieces, it turns out that most people's headaches cannot so easily be segregated into tension-type on the one hand and migraine-type on the other. Characteristics of certain headaches merge, blend and overlap with those of others. What starts out as neck stiffness in the morning turns into throbbing pain in your temples or behind one eye by afternoon, associated with nausea, photophobia, blurred vision and trouble concentrating, representing progressive activation of migraine. Or, during a month of more-frequent-than-usual severe headaches, you also have more mild-to-moderate, nonspecific background head and neck discomfort.

This is how we experience the broad and changing spectrum of migraine. It arises from a single mechanism, but since the degree of activation fluctuates, it is expressed to varying extents and in many different ways. Doctors often respond to patients with these multiple, overlapping complaints by diagnosing "mixed tension/vascular" headache. ("Vascular" is a synonym of "migraine.") This diagnosis implies that two separate headache-generating mechanisms are somehow acting simultaneously. The frequency with which "mixed" headache is diagnosed raises an obvious question: Is this a remarkable, recurring coincidence of two separate problems, or does the routine coexistence of multiple headache types point to a single underlying mechanism? You know the correct answer.

When people diagnosed with tension or mixed headache *do* improve with treatment, it's usually because the treatment happens to be effective for *migraine* or has nonspecific benefit. For instance, a doctor who suspects that depression is the cause of headache may prescribe a tricyclic antidepressant, and it may work . . . not because depression is the problem, but because a tricyclic antidepressant can help prevent migraine. Or, so-called muscle relaxants such as carisoprodol (Soma) and cyclobenzaprine (Flexeril), prescribed for presumed muscle tension, are really just mild sedatives that might relax you enough to lessen the stress component of your migraine trigger load or help you fall

"No matter what I did, my headaches kept coming back"

PATTY'S STORY

P atty had bought into the diagnosis of tension headache—
hook, line and sinker. After all, her headaches were *worse*
when she was stressed out, and she felt so much better
*(for a while) after a massage, a chiropractic treatment, a physical
therapy session, acupuncture, biofeedback or many of the other
temporarily soothing approaches that had failed to control her
headaches long-term.*

*And since she couldn't run off and get a massage every time her
head and neck hurt, Patty was glad she had her Imitrex to get her
through the day, even though she worried that taking it nearly
every day might be a bit too much.*

*Finally, Patty's husband insisted she see me. Patty was a hard
sell, especially when it came to giving up her Imitrex. But she did
it, and she followed the diet, and lo and behold: she has finally
controlled her headaches by discarding the misdiagnosis of tension
headache and following the 1-2-3 Program.* ◆

asleep, and so you feel better. You can see how, in these ways, inadvertent treatment success perpetuates the myth of tension headache and distracts from recognition of migraine as the real problem.

The Myth of Sinus Headache

CONSIDER THIS: the mucous membranes that line your nose and sinuses are chock-full of blood vessels. When migraine causes blood vessels around your head to become swollen and inflamed, its favorite targets include your nose and sinuses. The swelling and inflammation of blood vessels there produces congestion, pressure, stuffiness, postnasal drip, and pain: a so-called "sinus headache."

But you and your doctor don't realize that this is migraine. Instead, you suspect some allergy, infection or structural abnormality afflicting your sinuses. These conditions can indeed cause sinus symptoms, but so does migraine. *Big-time.*

Misdiagnosing Allergic Headache

AN ALLERGY is an overreaction of your immune system to a particular stimulus, such as inhaled pollen, a medication or something you eat. Allergies can produce many symptoms, including skin rash, itchy eyes, stuffy nose, scratchy throat and sneezing, but the common presumption that they can also cause substantial headaches is groundless. Yet it's amazing how many of my headache patients have previously been labeled with "allergic rhinitis" (rhinitis is nasal inflammation) or "allergic sinusitis" to account, at least in part, for their headaches.

People with so-called sinus headaches who undergo skin or blood testing for allergies often have positive test responses, which may lead to the false conclusion that their headaches have an allergic basis. Yes, you might develop welts when certain foreign substances are injected under your skin, or you may have certain antibodies in your blood. But translating these findings into an explanation for *headaches* takes a long leap of (senseless) faith.

Some common experiences further confuse the picture and reinforce the unfortunate myth of allergic headaches. When headaches are triggered by eating certain foods or by smelling perfumes, tobacco smoke or cleaning products, we tend to assume—sort of understandably, though incorrectly—that an allergic mechanism is involved. (Many people also assume that the association of headaches with barometric pressure changes, as when storms approach, implies allergy, but the logic of that escapes me.) In fact, these are all *migraine* triggers, and the mechanism of migraine is not that of allergy. Migraine triggers do not act by stimulating overreaction of your immune system, as do allergic triggers.

Matters are made worse when allergy medication seems to help headaches. Allergy or "sinus" medications often contain a decongestant. Decongestants constrict blood vessels, thereby temporarily relieving blood vessel swelling—including that due to migraine—and reducing congestion and pain behind your face. (Actually, when used regularly, decongestants cause rebound and insidiously make things worse long-term, as discussed in Chapter Three.) Nasal steroid sprays to treat presumed allergic problems act nonspecifically to alleviate inflammation of blood vessels in the sinuses—whether allergy or migraine is the cause—but favorable response to steroid sprays is likely to be misinterpreted as specific evidence that an allergy is at work.

Misdiagnosing Sinus Infection

NO QUESTION: acute bacterial infection of an obstructed sinus cavity can cause pain, usually accompanied by fever and pus-like nasal discharge. But the notion that *chronic, recurrent* infection is a common basis for *chronic, recurrent* sinus-type headache is nonsense. The true underlying mechanism? Migraine. When you think your escalating facial pain is due to a "sinus infection" that then secondarily triggers a "migraine," think again. You're overlooking the fact that migraine, revving up progressively, is the single culprit.

A common source of confusion is nose or sinus cultures showing the presence of bacteria that can cause infection. As it turns out, these bacteria normally live peacefully in the nose and sinuses of many people, colonizing the area but not causing infection. Suppose you're one of these people, and you experience a headache as a result of migraine producing swelling and inflammation of blood vessels in your nose and sinuses. Further suppose that a bacterial culture is performed. If the findings are positive, they are likely to be misconstrued as evidence that a sinus infection is causing your headache, even if the findings reflect only normal bacterial colonization.

The coincidence of a positive culture and pain too often adds up to the misdiagnosis of sinus infection, even in the absence of the expected hallmarks of infection: fever and pus-like nasal discharge. Frequently, sinus infection is (mis)diagnosed based on pain *alone*—pain that is actually due to migraine—without *either* clinical evidence of infection *or* positive culture results. In this scenario, when you improve while being treated with antibiotics, it isn't because the antibiotics are treating an infection; it's because a flare-up of unrecognized migraine has settled down on its own. But the mistaken notion that infection was the problem is reinforced.

Further confusion arises when migraine *causes* sinus infection. Here's how that works. Swelling of blood vessels due to migraine can cause swelling of the mucous membranes lining the narrow openings that drain your sinus cavities. When drainage becomes obstructed, bacteria that normally colonize your sinus cavities can overgrow and cause infection with pain, fever and nasal discharge. In this case, infection is usually diagnosed (correctly), and the symptoms of infection subside in response to antibiotics. Instead of recognizing the infection as an event resulting from the underlying problem of migraine, the infection is interpreted (incorrectly) as evidence of an underlying problem of chronic infection, a presumed smoldering volcano that erupts visibly from time to time.

On MCS

There are people who claim hypersensitivity to all sorts of environmental stimuli—who can't tolerate breathing air that's been in contact with a wide array of everyday things. They imprison themselves in "bubbles" of isolation in order to escape the ubiquitous "poisons" that lurk in the breeze; when they do go out, they wear masks for protection.

These *multiple chemical sensitivity* sufferers believe they have a super-duper allergy problem that causes their severe (over)reactions, including headaches. I've seen a number of these individuals as patients, and their headaches were triggered (in part) by odorants. But the perfumes, smoke and cleaning products that gave them headaches were triggering the migraine mechanism rather than acting upon some unique vulnerability. ◆

Radiologists inadvertently contribute to this tendency to misdiagnose migraine as sinus infection. Too often, imaging studies of the sinuses, including X rays and computed tomographic (CT) and magnetic resonance imaging (MRI) scans, show swelling of mucous membranes or obstructed drainage. The radiologist (mis)interprets these findings as "sinusitis," which leads your doctor to assume that you have an infection and to then treat you with antibiotics and decongestants. When your sinus symptoms improve—in response to the temporary blood vessel-constricting effect of decongestants, or because migraine has subsided spontaneously—the belief that recurrent infection is the problem is strengthened.

Let me clarify. The term "sinusitis" applied to this scenario is accurate, but it's also misleading. The suffix "itis" simply means inflammation, so migraine-related inflammation of blood vessels in the sinuses can be referred to as sinusitis. The problem is that in common usage sinusitis implies infection, which leads to reflexive (but in this case inappropriate) treatment with antibiotics and decongestants.

Misdiagnosing a Sinus Structural Abnormality

BESIDES ALLERGY AND INFECTION, a common explanation for sinus headache is a structural abnormality. For instance, blockage of one or more sinus cavities by an anatomical deformity is presumed to create a difference between the atmospheric pressure inside as compared with outside the cavity, somehow leading to pain. Or, pain is purported to result from the presence of a polyp or cyst, or a deviated nasal septum pressing against something.

The concept that a relatively stable structural abnormality could produce episodic severe pain stands on shaky ground. Why should a fixed structural abnormality cause severe headaches at some times but little or none at others? Why do *so* many people with sizable sinus polyps, cysts and nasal septal deviations (noted incidentally on X rays or other imaging studies) live without *any* substantial pain or other sinus symptoms? And why do so many headache patients who've had sinus surgery get no relief?

When people do respond favorably to sinus surgery for headaches, the response is often temporary. Within months if not weeks, their headaches return, sometimes in a different manner or with a vengeance. Temporary relief of headaches following sinus surgery can be explained in several ways. First, the placebo effect: one-third of people taking a sugar pill for pain will have temporary relief. The placebo effect is even more powerful when you've agreed to invasive surgery; you have a *strong* emotional investment that you've made the right decision.

What's in a Name?

An ironic exception to the general rule that sinusitis implies infection is the term "*vasomotor*" sinusitis (or *rhinitis*). "Vaso" refers to blood vessels, and "motor" indicates a disturbance of their regulation. The term, used mainly by ear, nose and throat specialists, describes blood vessel swelling and inflammation in the mucous membranes of the nose and sinuses for which there is no clear evidence of allergy or infection as the cause.

Where's the irony? The term "*vasomotor*" sinusitis (or *rhinitis*) correctly identifies the features of *migraine*: swelling of blood vessels and inflammation of the sinuses and nose. Migraine is the cause, but it's unrecognized as such and consequently untreated. ◆

Second, surgical removal of mucous membranes eliminates some of the target tissue within which migraine produces blood vessel swelling and inflammation. As a result, there is (temporarily) less opportunity for the mechanism of migraine to express itself . . . although migraine will eventually find its way to alternative target sites.

Third, sinus surgery that improves drainage can actually help migraine sufferers. Episodic blockage of sinus drainage (in this case due to migraine-related swelling of blood vessels in the mucous membranes) is less likely to occur if the drainage channels are surgically enlarged. Having said this, it's wiser to treat the primary underlying problem—migraine— than to do a plumbing job that won't hold up for very long. As long as migraine persists, one drain or another is likely to become clogged again.

"Six operations haven't fixed my sinus problem"

≈≈≈

MIGUEL'S STORY

By the time I saw him, Miguel had had not one, not two, not three, four or five, but six sinus operations—all to treat his headaches. Not to mention five years of allergy shots and countless medications, including all sorts of antibiotics, decongestants, antihistamines, steroids and you name it. Needless to say, the operations, shots and medications were all for naught.

All Miguel had to do to get rid of most of his headaches was to stop using the over-the-counter decongestants (Afrin spray and Sudafed tablets) from which he was rebounding and follow the diet. The relatively mild headaches that remained virtually vanished when he added verapamil for migraine prevention. It turned out that verapamil made him too constipated, so he switched to diltiazem and has been fine ever since. ◆

The Marketplace of Sinus Headache

Look closely at advertisements for sinus medications. Pay attention to the descriptions of throbbing, sickening pain, and notice the suffering, nauseated, photophobic faces depicted. Then tell me these poor souls aren't experiencing migraine.

Imagine how much money is spent on (and made from) these and other drugs, including expensive antibiotics and steroid sprays, prescribed for so-called sinus headache. Add the costs of allergy shots and sinus surgery for headaches. The expenditures (and profits) are staggering, as is the needless suffering, if these efforts are, as I believe, misguided attempts to treat problems that stem from migraine.

Don't misunderstand me. I'm not suggesting that the myth and misdiagnosis of sinus headache are part of a sinister plot. Conventional wisdom is the culprit. Healthcare enterprises are merely responding to the demands of the marketplace. The problem is that in this case the marketplace is a crowded bazaar that sells false goods. You can get a great deal on some emperor's clothes there. ◆

Summing Up

THE MISDIAGNOSES of allergy, infection and structural abnormality as causes of sinus headaches—and the treatments for these misdiagnoses—are not only mixed up to begin with but often mixed *together* in a further confusing jumble. Allergy and structural abnormality are said to lead to infection; allergy and infection are said to cause structural abnormalities such as polyps; and on and on. Over the years, so-called sinus headache sufferers are treated with innumerable courses of antihistamines, decongestants, steroid sprays, antibiotics, allergy shots, sinus irrigation and sinus surgery. Yet, despite accumulation of treatment failure, the stubborn myth (and misdiagnosis) of sinus headache lives on, and the real problem—migraine—goes unrecognized and untreated.

CHAPTER SEVEN

A Morass
of Misdiagnoses

Tension headache and sinus headache may be the most prevalent headache myths, but they have plenty of bad company. Let's explore some other common falsehoods in the diagnosis of headache.

Cervical Spine Disease

ABOUT HALF THE ADULTS who undergo X rays, CT scans or MRI scans of the neck turn out to have bone spurs and worn-down, bulging disks. In the vast majority of cases, these routine degenerative changes cause no symptoms whatsoever. When they do, the symptoms are predominately in the arms and hands. If a spinal nerve root on its way to your arm and hand is irritated or compressed, you may experience numbness, tingling, pain or weakness—but primarily in the arm and hand, *not* in the neck and head.

It's human nature to try to understand things, including headaches, based on what we can see and feel. If your doctor sees degenerative changes on imaging studies of your cervical spine, and you feel pain in your head associated with neck ache, stiffness and tenderness (which your doctor may be able to reproduce by pressing on your neck), it's tempting to add two and two and be confident that the answer is four. But if two and two don't have anything to do with each other, they don't add up to anything.

When neck symptoms are associated with chronic headaches, the cause of both is usually migraine. Migraine commonly causes discomfort not only in the head but also in and around the neck, including stiffness, aching, pressure, soreness, heaviness, tightness, "knots" and "spasm." Most people with both neck and head pain assume that muscle tension or some other problem with the spine, such as a pinched nerve in the neck, gives rise to pain in the neck that somehow spreads to the head, rather than realizing that migraine generates pain in both areas.

Remember, the cervical nerves, which are an integral part of the mechanism of migraine, travel in and around the neck. The territory of migraine extends even beyond the head and neck into what you might call your "shoulders"—actually, the trapezius muscles, which lie between the neck and shoulder joints—as well as into your shoulder blades. The discomfort that migraine generates in these regions is often chronic, experienced day in and day out.

The "muscular" quality of the discomfort, and the way it seems to relate to certain ways you sit or bend, reinforces the misconception that cervical spine disease or a pinched nerve, rather than migraine, is the source of pain. But if you recall that neck discomfort due to migraine stems in part from inflammation of blood vessels in the meninges, the membranes that line the brain and the spinal cord, you can begin to understand how migraine can be the source. Meningeal inflammation causes neck stiffness and pain *especially* when you flex your neck and thereby stretch the meninges, as when you're reading or working at a computer.

Did You Sleep the Wrong Way?

When we wake up with neck pain and headache, we tend to ascribe it to "sleeping the wrong way" and thereby getting a "crick" in the neck or pinching a nerve.

Well, maybe. Or maybe it has nothing at all to do with sleeping positions and instead has everything to do with migraine, which *often* causes pain on awakening. It may be caused by the overnight wearing off of the previous day's rebound-causing quick fix or dietary caffeine. Or migraine can be linked to the master clock in the brain, so that it's set off by a triggering influence that's preprogrammed to occur while we sleep or around the time we would otherwise wake up, like an alarm.

Sleep apnea is another consideration. This condition, in which pauses in breathing occur during sleep, can cause headaches (by triggering migraine?) and is especially likely in overweight men (and postmenopausal women) who snore loudly and are sleepy during the day. Sleep apnea can be diagnosed with a sleep study and treated with a special mask that delivers pressurized air during sleep.

Otherwise, if that special pillow you bought doesn't prevent you from waking with neck pain and headache, think migraine and try the 1-2-3 Program. ◆

The *nature* of certain activities, rather than the posture in which they're performed, can also cause headache. For instance, tasks such as reading and working at a computer can trigger migraine by virtue of the visual effort and mental concentration involved. In this case, it's a mistake to conclude that your position at your desk or workstation, by aggravating some problem in your neck, is causing your headache.

And so it is that symptoms of migraine are often mistakenly attributed to cervical spine disease. In some people, however, cervical spine disease may actually *trigger* migraine, thereby producing discomfort in and around the neck that is not *directly* caused by the underlying spinal problem. In other words, problems with your neck may activate sensory nerves that carry signals, which act as triggers, to the migraine control center in the brain. In this way, sensory impulses arising from problems in the neck may translate into head and neck pain *indirectly*, through the mechanism of migraine.

Confusing? Maybe, but this proposed neural circuit would explain several aspects of the relationship between migraine and neck symptoms. Therapeutic measures including neck massage, local heat, ultrasound, electrical stimulation, and manipulation may temporarily suppress sensory input tending to trigger migraine, thereby interrupting this circuit and relieving the discomfort that results.

Similarly, anesthetics injected around nerves in the neck or at the back of the head can temporarily relieve neck discomfort from migraine by blocking the triggering signals carried by these nerves to the migraine control center in the brain. Such injections may also block nerves on the output side of the migraine mechanism; that is, nerves carrying impulses that would lead to blood vessel swelling and inflammation (and thereby cause pain) may be blocked by an anesthetic as well.

You might wonder: if a musculoskeletal problem in the neck *is* triggering migraine, why not just fix the problem? To begin with, the findings of neck X rays or MRI scans may *look* like problems but usually *aren't*; they're just there, inconsequentially. Or, even if a problem is genuine and is triggering migraine, trying to fix it may be risky or unreliable. Be wary of cervical spine surgery directed at pain predominately in the head and neck as opposed to the radiating arm pain that characterizes a truly symptomatic cervical disk. Cervical spine surgery for headaches and neck pain is likely to be aimed at the *wrong* target, when the *right* target is migraine.

Neck Noise

A curious feature of migraine is what people describe as cracking, creaking, crunching, grinding or popping in the neck. Doctors routinely attribute this to "arthritis," but these cracking and popping feelings tend to come and go in concert with discomfort, which makes sense if *migraine* is the culprit. Unlike degenerative arthritis, migraine naturally fluctuates. In addition, many individuals with cracking and creaking have *no* evidence of arthritis in the neck on X rays or CT or MRI scans.

Of course, it's not *always* migraine when someone's neck cracks. Still, if your head and neck often hurt, and when they hurt your neck cracks a lot, to me that's migraine. I don't know *how* migraine causes these noises in your neck. But as much as I think I do know about migraine, there's a whole lot more that I know I *don't* know. ◆

Short of surgery, many other treatments are directed at cervical spine disease and similar problems mistakenly presumed to be sources of headaches and neck pain. Among these treatments are physical therapy, osteopathic manipulation, chiropractic, therapeutic massage, acupuncture, biofeedback, electrical stimulation, trigger-point injections, nerve blocks and epidural steroid injections. Sometimes these approaches provide relief of symptoms—temporarily, at least—even when the underlying problem is migraine. That could be because they've suppressed nerve impulses that would otherwise feed into a reverberating loop of migraine. But don't underestimate the placebo effect, and the powerful therapeutic benefit of close contact with a caring person, which characterizes most "alternative" approaches.

Posttraumatic Headache and Postconcussive Syndrome

POSTTRAUMATIC HEADACHE is simply headache that follows a blow to or a jarring of the head. Head trauma of this type may result in vexing headaches, even without apparent injury to the skull, brain or cervical spine. Other symptoms of so-called posttraumatic or postconcussive syndrome include dizziness, unsteadiness, vertigo, blurred vision, tinnitus, trouble concentrating . . . in other words, a generous assortment of migraine symptoms. To a large extent, posttraumatic headache and postconcussive syndrome *are* migraine. (I've often wondered how many athletes said to have "concussions" resulting in headaches and dizziness actually have posttraumatic migraine and could be effectively treated with the 1-2-3 Program.)

Blows to the head, without damaging the brain, can somehow lower the threshold for activation of migraine so that the threshold is crossed more easily (see Figure 13, page 154). Over time, usually within days, weeks or months, the threshold tends to drift back up to baseline. When headaches and other migraine symptoms linger long after traumatic onset, it's likely that some other factor—such as rebound or psychological pressures of personal injury litigation—is perpetuating the problem. The diagnosis of posttraumatic headache or postconcussive syndrome is a therapeutic dead end, leading to no specific treatment. Recognizing posttraumatic migraine, on the other hand, opens the door to effective therapy.

A twist on posttraumatic migraine is *postsurgical* migraine. Persistent headaches sometimes develop following surgery to remove benign tumors of the nerve that connects the ear to the brain (acoustic neuromas) as well as after other invasive procedures

Roller Coaster Headache

I love roller coasters. I'm a card-carrying enthusiast. (Really.) But once in a while I get a headache after a coaster ride. Other people I know do, too.

I finally figured out what was happening: these are short-lived versions of *posttraumatic migraine*, brought on by the jarring nature of amusement rides that shake your head (and brain) around quite a bit. Also, I've realized from listening to my patients that other physical activities—such as waterskiing or heading a soccer ball—can have the same temporary effect. Personally, I still ride coasters, because I love them enough to be willing to pay the relatively small price that may follow. ◆

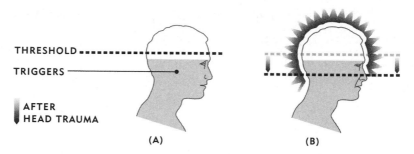

FIGURE 13: POSTTRAUMATIC MIGRAINE. *Before head trauma, the migraine mechanism remains inactive and there's no symptom (A). After trauma, the threshold falls below the trigger level (B) and active symptoms result.*

around the head. When there is no other reasonable explanation for these postoperative headaches, such as an infection or a fluid collection, the mechanism is migraine. It seems that some aspect of the physical trauma of surgery around the head can lower your threshold for migraine activation. A similar phenomenon occurs in some people who seemingly recover from meningitis (usually caused by a viral infection) yet have persistent problems with migraine in its wake.

Whiplash

WHIPLASH IS SUDDEN unintentional movement of the neck: usually backward, then forward, typically as a result of being rear-ended while sitting in a motor vehicle. Stretching and tearing of muscle and ligament fibers can occur, causing neck discomfort. This kind of soft tissue injury resolves spontaneously within a few weeks to months at most.

Individuals with *persistent* neck symptoms and headaches following whiplash-type injury often also suffer from posttraumatic migraine as a result of jarring of the head, although it is not usually recognized or treated. The failure to see this as part of the spectrum of migraine is another example of our natural tendency to think about pain in mechanical, musculoskeletal terms . . . combined with our unquestioning acceptance of the narrow conventional definition of migraine.

"They told me I was brain-damaged!"

ANDREA'S STORY

I t didn't seem like such a big deal at the time. Andrea's car was rear-ended, and her head may have bumped against something (she was briefly dazed), but she never expected the ensuing aftermath of seemingly endless headaches and neck pain.

Andrea tried physical therapy and had a series of "trigger point" injections into her neck; neither helped long-term. Midrin, a quick-fix medication, worked for a few hours at a time, so she took it several times a day. Meanwhile, she felt more and more forgetful and discouraged.

Andrea's lawyer in the accident case sent her to a neuropsychologist, who tested her (while she had a bad headache, which was very distracting, and was taking her medication, which made her "spacey") and diagnosed traumatic brain injury. Her spirits plummeted when she heard she was "damaged goods" and might not recover.

A friend sent Andrea to me, and her free fall ended. I explained that her brain had not been injured, and that the neuropsychologist's diagnosis was an overblown, litigation-driven (mis)interpretation of some minor test findings attributable to her psychological state and medication side effects. What she had was posttraumatic migraine, complicated by rebound from Midrin and emotional turmoil.

Andrea did very well by following the 1-2-3 Program and resolving her lawsuit. In the long run, her headaches subsided to her natural baseline, which she has controlled readily with partial dietary modification alone. ◆

Trigeminal Neuralgia and Atypical Facial Pain

TRIGEMINAL NEURALGIA (that is, trigeminal nerve pain) is very distinctive: severe, sudden, brief, electric shock–like pains on one side of the face, typically triggered by lightly touching or otherwise stimulating the face or mouth while washing, chewing or toothbrushing. Usually it occurs in older people, probably because a small blood vessel is rubbing against the trigeminal nerve just before it enters the brain stem, but it can also occur in younger people—sometimes as a result of a benign tumor or multiple sclerosis. Trigeminal neuralgia is a straightforward diagnosis, clearly distinguishable from migraine.

But migraine often *does* produce various kinds of pain in the face, different from the pain that characterizes trigeminal neuralgia. Among other differences, facial pain due to migraine (a) may be on both sides or may alternate sides, whereas trigeminal neuralgia is always on the same side, (b) is longer-lasting than the fleeting paroxysms of pain from trigeminal neuralgia, and (c) is not triggered by lightly touching the face or the other ways characteristic of trigeminal neuralgia.

Treatment of trigeminal neuralgia is relatively effective in most cases. Antiseizure medications such as carbamazepine (Tegretol), phenytoin (Dilantin) and gabapentin (Neurontin) are the first choices, and other medications as well as injections or surgery (to separate the nerve from any blood vessel that might be irritating it) are additional treatment options. *The message here is:* if facial pain isn't characteristic of trigeminal neuralgia and doesn't respond to adequate treatment for it, and if there isn't a clear alternative explanation such as acute bacterial sinusitis or an abscessed tooth, the cause is probably migraine. The all-too-frequent diagnosis of "atypical facial pain" is nothing but a wastebasket diagnosis that leads nowhere in terms of treatment and belongs in the wastebasket itself.

Occipital Neuralgia

OCCIPITAL NEURALGIA is a diagnosis meant to account for pain, numbness, tingling or other abnormal sensations over one side of the back of the head, presumably caused by an irritation or compression of the occipital nerve as it travels through a groove at the base of the skull. If that region has been substantially injured, resulting in major damage to or scarring of the nerve, the diagnosis of occipital neuralgia may be reasonable. But when pain, numbness, tingling or other abnormal sensation occurs spontaneously, *without* substantial direct trauma to the nerve, think migraine. (A common error is to diagnose occipital neuralgia following whiplash-type injury, rather than recognizing the routine occurrence of posttraumatic migraine in that setting.)

The occipital nerves derive from cervical nerves and interact with neighboring blood vessels in the migraine mechanism to produce local pain, numbness, tingling or other abnormal sensations. These include sensations such as burning, prickling, water trickling, pins and needles, or vibration, and often the occipital nerves are tender to the touch. If you respond well to occipital nerve blocks, your doctor is likely to misinterpret your response as confirmation of the diagnosis of occipital neuralgia, even though your response is caused simply by interruption of outgoing and incoming nerve impulses along this particular pathway of migraine.

Temporomandibular Joint (TMJ) Dysfunction and Dental Problems

TMJ DYSFUNCTION can produce pain, tenderness, clicking, slipping, locking or restricted motion of the jaw joints. Too often, however, symptoms beyond the territory of the jaw joints but within the realm of migraine, such as headache and neck pain, are mistakenly attributed to TMJ or some other "bite" problem and are (mis)treated with physical therapy, soft diets, bite plates, injections of anesthetics and steroids, and even jaw joint surgery.

These measures may be reasonable for symptoms *clearly* caused by mechanical TMJ dysfunction but are misguided when the symptoms are those of migraine, as when head pain is neither focused in the

---

"That car accident ruined my life"

≈≈

YOLANDA'S STORY

I never actually treated Yolanda. We met when I examined her and reviewed her records at the request of an insurance company that she was suing after a car accident. Following a series of occipital nerve blocks, some of which had seemed to temporarily reduce her post-accident headaches and neck pain, she'd undergone occipital nerve ablation: a procedure to more permanently deaden the nerves that were thought to have been injured so as to cause her pain.

It didn't work. In fact, Yolanda's pain was worse than ever. So, next she had an operation on a bulging disk in her neck, which didn't work, either. All the while she was gobbling painkillers like candy and going down the drain, physically and emotionally.

Why? Because she suffered from undiagnosed and untreated posttraumatic migraine—not injury to her occipital nerves or a cervical disk—and she was rebounding to beat the band. Not to mention her vested interest in being a victim by virtue of her litigation: the worse she was, the better off she was in terms of a potentially big payoff. It's really unfortunate, but it happens. All too often. ◆

jaw joints nor strongly associated with jaw opening or chewing. The diagnosis of TMJ dysfunction has even been stretched to account for neurological symptoms such as dizziness, tinnitus and blurred vision—symptoms that are well explained by migraine but difficult to reckon on the basis of mechanical dysfunction of the jaw joints.

Dental problems apart from TMJ dysfunction—such as malocclusion (a misaligned bite) or a hidden abscess—are sometimes implicated and treated as causes of chronic headaches. When a dental problem *is* painful, the pain is focal (at its origin) and the problem is usually self-evident: it hurts like heck when you bite down on it. Migraine doesn't do that, but it can produce pain predominately in your teeth or jaw, and it's *certainly* a more likely cause of pain elsewhere around your head, face or neck than some vague, elusive, can't-quite-put-your-finger-on-it dental problem. Think twice—no, make that three times—before having extensive dental work done to treat your headaches.

Fibromyalgia and Myofascial Pain Dysfunction

THESE LABELS are among those applied to chronic, diffuse pain that defies clear explanation. When otherwise unexplained pain is mainly in or around the head, face or neck (including the trapezius muscle and shoulder blade regions), *migraine*—a *treatable* condition (unlike these dead-end diagnoses)—is likely.

Chronic Fatigue Syndrome (CFS), Neurally Mediated Hypotension (NMH) and Arnold-Chiari Malformation

CFS, ANOTHER CONTROVERSIAL diagnosis, describes tiredness that can't be accounted for on the basis of an identifiable physical problem, although some doctors claim there is a physical problem: NMH. This diagnosis often arises from tilt-table testing, a "provocative," non-physiological method of testing in which you're strapped upright,

Can Large Breasts Cause Headaches?

No, of course not, but over the years I've cared for about a half-dozen women who had previously undergone breast-reduction surgery in the hope of relieving their headaches. They assumed (or were talked into believing) that the downward pull of excessive breast tissue caused poor posture, with hunching of the neck and shoulders, and consequently headaches. Needless to say, postoperatively their headaches continued unabated.

As much as I sympathize with each one of my patients who has suffered needlessly because of headache misdiagnosis and mistreatment, my heart aches especially for these unwitting victims of their own sheer desperation and the mind-boggling foolishness of their doctors. ◆

with no support for your legs, waiting to see if you get dizzy after too long. Tilt-table testing is fraught with false-positive errors, meaning that the findings are unrelated to any problem in the real world. Not surprisingly, because these people aren't much different from the rest of us, headaches (due to unrecognized, untreated migraine) often occur in individuals labeled with CFS and NMH.

A recent twist on the diagnoses of CFS and NMH is the suggestion that they are somehow related to Arnold-Chiari malformation: a congenital anatomical deformity in which the lower parts of the brain lie *too* low and can cause crowding at the base of the skull and, uncommonly as a result, problems due to compression of the brain stem. The large majority of people with this finding on MRI scans have no problem from it; it's an "incidental" finding. But some neurosurgeons have offered a "cure" for CFS by operating on the malformation to relieve alleged "pressure" from it that ostensibly is leading to NMH (and in turn headaches, which instead are actually due to unrecognized, untreated migraine).

Let the buyer beware. Rather than surrendering your headaches to the clutches of the diagnosis of CFS, or subjecting yourself to needless surgery for Arnold-Chiari malformation, why not give the 1-2-3 Program a chance?

Systemic Lupus Erythematosus

CALLED LUPUS FOR SHORT, this disorder of the immune system can lead to damage of many organ systems, including the skin, joints, kidneys and brain. A blood test for antinuclear antibodies (ANA) is one of the basic elements of diagnosing lupus, but this test is often falsely positive: the level is elevated in many people who don't have the disease.

What does this have to do with migraine? Well, I've seen many patients diagnosed with lupus—some with legitimate disease and others who were probably misdiagnosed because of a falsely positive ANA (a very common result)—who have had headaches due not to lupus but to migraine yet were being treated for presumed "active" lupus without any other evidence of disease activity. This is no small problem, not only because the medications for lupus aren't right for migraine—and so the headaches persist, and treatment is further mistakenly escalated—but also because these medications have potentially serious side effects.

Giant Cell (Temporal) Arteritis

HERE'S ANOTHER CONDITION that is diagnosed largely on the basis of a blood test (sedimentation rate) that is often falsely positive, so that the condition is sometimes (mis)diagnosed when it's not really present. In GCA the immune system attacks blood vessels around the head and thereby causes headaches, usually in older people. It can also cause loss of vision, so you don't want to miss the diagnosis, especially since corticosteroid treatment is highly effective.

But you also don't want to make the diagnosis of GCA *incorrectly* and thereby subject someone to unnecessary, potentially dangerous

Do You Have Lyme Disease?

Lyme disease is real. It's an infectious disease acquired when you're bitten by a contaminated deer tick, and it can cause problems including rash, flu-like illness, and arthritis. There can even be neurological involvement, usually in the form of temporary weakness of one side of the face (facial palsy) which, like the rest of Lyme's afflictions, responds readily to antibiotic treatment.

Rarely, Lyme disease infects the brain and thereby can cause a host of neurological symptoms—but *not* primarily headaches. Yet I've seen a bunch of headache patients who've been convinced that their chronic headaches (and forgetfulness, and fatigue, and so on) stem from persistent Lyme disease.

Some of these people *did* once have Lyme disease (with characteristic clinical pictures and positive blood tests), but they were long ago cured by appropriate therapy and their ongoing headaches relate to *migraine*. Some of them just won't buy this, despite overwhelming evidence— including normal MRI scans— that their brains were *never* involved by the disease.

I've even seen a few patients who probably never did have Lyme disease (they never had the characteristic picture or positive blood tests) but who were nonetheless diagnosed with it and treated with *endless courses of intravenous antibiotics* (at huge expense and with considerable risk) all because of chronic headaches due to unrecognized, untreated *migraine*! It's *scary*. ◆

treatment. Over the years I've seen at least two dozen people who have suffered this fate. Biopsy of the temporal arteries can confirm the diagnosis of GCA, but in these cases either it wasn't done or the biopsy results were negative yet were assumed to be *falsely* negative . . . rather than recognizing that the blood test was falsely *positive*.

It's a tricky situation, because steroids can relieve headaches not only from GCA but also from migraine! And so these individuals felt better on steroids—because the treatment relieved undiagnosed migraine, not misdiagnosed GCA—and their improvement reinforced the misdiagnosis. When they tried to reduce the dosage of steroids, they felt worse (as people often do when withdrawing from steroids, taken for any purpose), and this provided further misguidance. In the end, these folks would have been better off if they hadn't had the blood test in the first place.

Hypoglycemia

TRUE HYPOGLYCEMIA (low blood sugar) is uncommon, but the diagnosis of hypoglycemia often is improperly applied to headaches, nausea, dizziness and lightheadedness: symptoms of migraine. Many of my patients with migraine were told in the past that they suffer from hypoglycemia and were advised to eat frequent small meals. That may not be bad advice, insofar as waiting too long between meals can trigger migraine, but the diagnosis of hypoglycemia is usually a misdiagnosis. Don't be fooled by minor abnormalities—insignificant findings, really—of glucose tolerance tests used to diagnose hypoglycemia. This is another good example of test results *clouding* rather than *clarifying* the diagnostic picture, and why tests should be obtained only when *clearly* indicated.

Eyestrain

EYESTRAIN IS A POPULAR but fuzzy concept that associates visual and mental tasks (such as reading or using a computer) with visual blurring and discomfort in the eyes and around the head. Many chronic headache sufferers have sought relief by having their eyes checked and getting new corrective lenses, to no avail. No wonder: they're barking up the wrong tree. Remember that *migraine* can be triggered by

Blood Tests for Headaches?

In selected patients, a few tests *might* be reasonable: complete blood counts (CBCs) to check for anemia and thyroid stimulating hormone (TSH) to rule out hyperthyroidism— both of which can trigger migraine—and an erythrocyte sedimentation rate (ESR) to screen for giant cell arteritis in certain older individuals.

What is *not* appropriate is to routinely send off all sorts of other blood tests looking for lupus, Lyme disease, vitamin B_{12} deficiency and a host of other conditions that are *not* causes of staightforward chronic headaches. But it's done all the time, and too often one of these tests will ring a bell: a false alarm. ◆

visual effort and mental concentration, thereby causing visual blurring and discomfort in your eyes and around your head— which you might mistakenly suspect to be eyestrain.

Eustachian Tube Dysfunction

MIGRAINE PRODUCES swelling of blood vessels in mucous membranes around your head and gives rise to congestion and discomfort that not only are misdiagnosed as sinus headache but also can affect the ears. The eustachian tubes, which connect the middle ear with the back of the nose, are lined by mucous membranes. If migraine causes blood vessels in these mucous membranes to swell, resulting in engorgement of the mucous membranes, the eustachian tubes can become blocked.

The result is ear discomfort: fullness, stuffiness, pressure and pain. Additionally, when blockage of the eustachian tubes leads to a pressure differential between the two sides of the eardrum, the eardrum is pushed away from the side of higher pressure. And that hurts even more! But treating ear pain arising from migraine with antibiotics and decongestants for a phantom ear infection is foolish. Be suspicious of the recurrent diagnosis of ear infection in adults; it's usually a misdiagnosis of what is really migraine.

"Blood thinners did nothing for my headaches"

INGRID'S STORY

Ingrid had suffered persistent headaches for four months, ever since an episode of sudden, severe headache with visual blurring and numbness that started in her left hand and spread to her left arm, leg and tongue over a period of several minutes. She also briefly felt forgetful, confused and unsteady, and her speech was slightly garbled.

Ingrid had lots and lots of tests. One was positive for antiphospholipid antibodies, which can produce a syndrome in which people suffer blood clots, miscarriages and strokes. But these antibodies are also present in many people who have no problem (like Ingrid's mother, who was symptom-free). Because Ingrid had symptoms, her doctors treated her with the standard approach: a potent blood thinner. Yet her headaches continued, as did episodes similar to (but milder than) the original one.

So Ingrid was sent my way. To me, the picture was clear: migraine. If the antibodies played any role, which I doubted, it was by somehow triggering migraine—and regardless, migraine was what needed to be treated. So what happened? I don't know. Ingrid didn't follow up with me, apparently because she was sold on the antibody syndrome diagnosis.

Was I right? Again, I don't know. But I hope she doesn't suffer a complication of the potentially dangerous medication she's on. And even in retrospect, I would never have ordered that blood test to begin with, because in Ingrid's case the likelihood of its being truly positive—indicative of the real problem at hand and therefore helpful—is so much less than the likelihood of being falsely positive and thereby harmful, despite best intentions. ◆

Accumulation of secretions resulting from migraine-related blockage of the eustachian tubes can produce a sensation of fluid in the ear, and hearing may become muffled. When blocked eustachian tubes temporarily open, you may hear popping or clicking sounds as air moves to equilibrate the pressures on either side of the eardrum. Who would have thought that migraine could be at the bottom of all this?

CHAPTER EIGHT

Misdiagnoses of "Non-Headache" Migraine

A s broad as the spectrum of migraine is, even broader is the range of misdiagnoses of migraine. These misdiagnoses involve not only the variety of headaches and other forms of migraine discomfort, as we've seen, but also its many non-headache symptoms.

Misdiagnoses of Autonomic Symptoms

GASTROINTESTINAL SYMPTOMS OF MIGRAINE such as nausea, vomiting, constipation and diarrhea are often regarded—mistakenly—as a primary GI problem instead of being seen as part of the migraine picture. Some people think their headaches result from constipation, not realizing that constipation and headaches can *both* arise from migraine, sometimes with constipation preceding and therefore seeming to lead to headache.

Occasionally, migraine-related skin changes such as flushing are misinterpreted as an allergy problem, or a skin disease, or a hormonal disorder. If you get a fever, you probably have an infection, but actual fever associated with migraine, without infection, is not that rare. (Feverish *feelings*, or chills, are *commonly* experienced with migraine, but usually without measurable abnormality of body temperature.)

Misdiagnoses of Visual Symptoms

BEYOND MISINTERPRETATION OF MIGRAINE as "eyestrain," there are many other frequent errors in diagnosing the visual disturbances of migraine. Used properly, the term "floaters" refers to small, faint gray specks that tend to be fairly constant and are seen best while staring at a bright white wall. Floaters represent shadows cast upon your retina by tiny particles floating within the fluid that fills your eyeball. Generally, they're not a cause for concern. Spots in your vision that are bright, colorful, lively or rapidly moving are *not* floaters—although they're frequently called that in error—and are much more likely to be visual symptoms of migraine.

In contrast, transient visual loss from a blood clot cutting off the blood flow to your eye is "negative" in nature, rather than "positive," as with migraine. For instance, you might see a dark curtain come down over the vision in one eye for a few minutes, as opposed to scintillating spots or flashing lights from migraine. Despite the obvious differences in symptoms, I've seen quite a few patients with clear-cut (to me) migraine visual disturbances who had received treatment for presumed blood clots, including potent blood thinners and carotid artery surgery!

Retinal detachment can cause sparkles or flashes of light similar to those seen with migraine, so it may be prudent to see an eye doctor the first time these symptoms appear. But the vast majority of fleeting visual disturbances as described above are due to migraine, whether or not accompanied by headache.

Misdiagnoses of Vestibular Symptoms

FAILURE TO APPRECIATE THE FREQUENCY with which migraine causes dizziness, unsteadiness and the spinning sensation called vertigo gives rise to all-too-frequent misdiagnoses such as "labyrinthitis" and "inner ear infection" (usually attributed to a virus) or "sinus" (which hardly makes any sense; it's quite a stretch from the sinuses to the inner ear). These "tried and true" explanations are largely tired and false. They offer no solution for the dizziness they supposedly cause. The common practice of prescribing meclizine (Antivert), which is nothing more than a mild, nonspecific sedative, may be of benefit to your doctor, who can claim to have done *something* for you when you're dizzy, but does nothing for you except to relax you or help you fall asleep. Two other frequent diagnoses of dizziness (specifically of vertigo) may be legitimate entities apart from migraine, or may belong at least in part to the spectrum of migraine: benign paroxysmal positional vertigo and Ménière's disease.

Many doctors think that psychological or emotional factors lie beneath chronic, recurrent dizziness: an explanation that lets them dodge the difficult question *Why can't I help these patients?* The answer is simple: *Because you're misdiagnosing them.* In most cases of otherwise unexplained dizziness, the correct diagnosis is migraine, which proper treatment—the 1-2-3 Program—can control.

Misdiagnoses of Somatosensory Symptoms

THE SOMATOSENSORY SYMPTOMS OF MIGRAINE, such as numbness and tingling, are usually fleeting, vague and nonspecific. Often, incorrect labels are attached to these symptoms. Anxiety, hyperventilation and

When Your Head Spins, Is It BPPV?

BPPV, or benign paroxysmal positional vertigo, is said to cause vertigo, nausea and unsteadiness that lasts seconds to minutes and occurs when your head is in a certain position, usually turned to one particular side when you're lying down. It is believed that BPPV results when tiny crystals in the inner ear break loose and float into one of the fluid-filled semicircular canals, the motion sensors in your inner ear. The presence of these crystals where they don't belong has an irritating effect, giving rise to a volley of abnormal signals traveling from the motion sensors to your brain. The brain interprets these signals as though you're spinning, and as a result you *feel* that you're spinning—even though you're not. There is treatment for BPPV: a series of head-positioning maneuvers designed to shift the offending crystals to a place in the inner ear where they won't cause trouble. And sometimes this works.

On the other hand, vertigo is also positional in patients with vestibular dysfunction due to migraine. This may be another example of sensory input (in this case, information about your head position derived from the semicircular canals) feeding into the circuit of migraine as a trigger. The association of migraine and motion sickness (such as car sickness, seasickness or intolerance of amusement rides) similarly reflects vestibular stimulation as a migraine trigger.

Posttraumatic BPPV following head trauma or whiplash-type injury is presumed to arise from traumatic dislocation of tiny crystals into one of the semicircular canals. Posttraumatic migraine, causing vestibular dysfunction with or without headaches, is an alternative (and in my experience more common) explanation for posttraumatic dizziness and vertigo.

I'll accept that there is an entity, BPPV, that exists apart from migraine, but I am convinced that much of what is *labeled* BPPV is migraine. The bottom line is: If treatment for BPPV doesn't get rid of your vertigo, consider—and treat—migraine. ◆

Or Could It Be Ménière's?

Ménière's disease (named for the French physician Prosper Ménière) is said to cause attacks lasting from minutes to hours and consisting of pressure, temporary hearing loss and tinnitus in one ear, along with vertigo, unsteadiness, nausea and sweating: a familiar constellation of *migraine* symptoms.

Without doubt, most of the patients I see who have been labeled with Ménière's disease suffer instead from migraine. The permanent low-frequency hearing loss that sometimes occurs after repeated episodes of so-called Ménière's may actually arise from damage to nerve cells in the inner ear as a result of migraine-related blood vessel constriction. Ménière's disease supposedly stems from episodic buildup of fluid pressure within the inner ear, but this may reflect the mechanism of migraine at work.

The response to conventional treatment of presumed Ménière's disease (using salt restriction and fluid pills) is often *under*whelming. As with benign paroxysmal positional vertigo (BPPV), many (if not all) individuals diagnosed with Ménière's suffer instead from migraine, for which proper preventive treatment—the 1-2-3 Program—has proven highly effective. ◆

panic attacks can cause numbness and tingling in the fingers or around the mouth that may be difficult to distinguish from similar effects of migraine. On the other hand, carpal tunnel syndrome, cervical nerve root irritation and peripheral neuropathy are neurological conditions with specific patterns of numbness and tingling that should not be confused with symptoms of migraine, but nonetheless they sometimes are.

Somatosensory symptoms that migrate within seconds or minutes over one side of the face or body may be misdiagnosed as seizures. At least several times a year I evaluate people with numbness and tingling—due to migraine but unrecognized as such—who have been told they have multiple sclerosis (MS) based partly on symptoms and partly on nonspecific, inconsequential findings—little bright spots—on MRI scans. (Such findings can also be associated with migraine, or most often are best regarded as just plain normal, since they're so common.) Ironically, these scans typically were ordered to provide reassurance that the individual didn't have a brain tumor, or whatever, but instead ended up creating a nightmare of anxiety.

"I've lived with vertigo for most of my life"

WILLARD'S STORY

For 30 years, as often as twice a week, Willard had been plagued by "Ménière's attacks" consisting of vertigo, sweating, nausea, vomiting, photophobia and imbalance. Six months before I met him, a new twist emerged: "mini attacks" with dizziness, unsteadiness and lightheadedness, but not true vertigo, and also with "pulsing, throbbing" right head pain—a brand-new feature.

Suspecting migraine (as the cause of the whole story, not just the recent symptoms), I counseled Willard about the migraine diet and advised his primary doctor to change his blood pressure medicine to verapamil. After four months, Willard was "better—not great, but better."

Six months later, having increased his verapamil dosage from 240 to 360 mg daily, he felt "much better." He was, in his own words, glad to have his life back . . . with no attacks, Ménière's, mini or otherwise. ◆

Misdiagnoses of Psychic and Emotional Symptoms

THE FREQUENT COEXISTENCE, mutual reinforcement and possible shared origins of migraine, depression and panic attacks can make it difficult to determine where each one stops and the others start. Mistakes are often made in failing to see that migraine, though increasingly active, is at least *part* of the story, if not the gist of it, when

"They said I had MS"

NATASHA'S STORY

T he report of Natasha's MRI scan had devastated her. What led to the scan was a month of recurrent numbness and tingling spreading from her right cheek to the back of her head, left arm and either leg, within minutes. Both the radiologist and her previous neurologist interpreted the scan, which showed several small bright spots, as indicative of multiple sclerosis.

Natasha imagined the worst: that she was doomed to wind up in a wheelchair. I'd like to think that I would have diagnosed migraine anyway—based on the characteristic fleeting nature of her sensory symptoms, wholly unlike the much more persistent symptoms of MS—but the diagnosis was all the more obvious with her long-standing history of constant head "pressure" (for which she took ibuprofen daily) and severe throbbing headaches, nausea and photophobia with her periods and after drinking red wine.

On the diet, her sensory symptoms resolved within a week. Because of persistent headaches, we added low-dose nortriptyline. Natasha's response: "My headaches are gone." Over the last several years, she's had only "a touch of numbness" when she fails to follow the diet carefully enough around her periods or when a storm approaches. ◆

Migraine and Anxiety

L et's say you experience new or increased symptoms of migraine, such as headaches, dizziness, or numbness and tingling. You go from doctor to doctor and have test after test. If the tests are normal, you become more and more frustrated, since you sense your doctor becoming more suspicious that it's "all in your head"even though you know *something* is wrong.

If some tests are abnormal, the results generate heightened anxiety that you *do* have *something*, despite the results being either nonspecifically abnormal (indicating no problem in particular), falsely positive (suggesting a problem that doesn't really exist) or

simply irrelevant. No one can seem to sort out what's wheat and what's chaff. Abnormal (but meaningless) test results coupled with failed, misguided treatments breed increased uncertainty, more and more tests and greater anxiety.

Of course, your anxiety (and lack of sleep) in turn stimulate your underlying, unrecognized problem of migraine; your migraine symptoms grow and grow; you become more and more focused on them, creating more anxiety and worse sleep, leading to escalating migraine symptoms . . . and so on in a classic vicious cycle. But because you've become a *complete nervous wreck*, it's easy to blame it all on you. ◆

depression or panic attacks mingle with headaches, dizziness, numbness and tingling, and other migraine symptoms. Instead, headaches, dizziness and these other symptoms are presumed to reflect psychological and emotional problems, and treatment is misdirected away from the easily hittable target of migraine. Similarly, migraine and anxiety reverberate, and as anxiety escalates, the accompanying presence of migraine becomes more and more obscured as this vicious cycle spins wildly into a maelstrom.

Confusion About Seizures

FOR STARTERS, migraine can trigger a seizure, and vice versa. But instances of migraine-related blood vessel constriction in the brain causing a seizure are very uncommon. Much more often, migraine—usually in the form of headache—occurs in the wake of a seizure.

Migraine is sometimes misdiagnosed as seizures, as when it causes numbness and tingling that spread over one side of the face or body. Another opportunity for misdiagnosis of seizures is when episodes of dizziness, confusion or loss of consciousness stem from migraine. Olfactory symptoms of migraine—specifically, smelling illusory odors—may be mistaken for seizure auras. I've seen dozens of new patients who have needlessly carried the dual burdens of a diagnosis of and treatment for seizures, but who really just have migraine.

Confusion About Stroke and Transient Ischemic Attacks

RARELY, MIGRAINE causes stroke. And because this is relatively rare, it may go unrecognized. People with stroke from migraine may be diagnosed with and treated for some other presumed cause, which is less than ideal when something could or should be done to avert further migraine trouble, not to mention the risks associated with (mis)treatment for the (mis)diagnosis of some other presumed cause of stroke. Confidence in the diagnosis of migraine-related stroke requires thoughtful evaluation by an experienced neurologist, with consideration of other reasonable possibilities.

Much more frequently, confusion between migraine and stroke relates to stroke-like episodes known as transient ischemic attacks (TIAs). TIAs are brief, symptomatic episodes of reduced blood flow (ischemia) affecting a specific part of the brain as a result of a blood

The EEG Example

The likelihood of mistaking migraine for seizures increases when migraine causes abnormal findings of electroencephalography (EEG), the recording of brain waves used as a diagnostic test for seizures. EEG findings are *often* nonspecific, may be abnormal in individuals with no neurologic problem and commonly are over-interpreted, especially as being indicative of seizures even when no such problem exists.

The likelihood of abnormal EEG findings is greater in individuals with highly active migraine, in whom the brain's electrical function may be abnormal at times. EEG findings of abnormal brain function due to migraine shouldn't be misconstrued as a seizure problem, but they sometimes are.

Be careful of even "noninvasive" EEG tests. They can hurt you. ◆

vessel being blocked temporarily, usually by a blood clot. The clot generally arises from one of the carotid arteries (the large arteries on either side of the neck that carry blood to the brain) or from the heart. Common symptoms of TIAs include numbness or weakness on one side of the body, loss of vision in one eye or difficulty in speaking, occurring suddenly and usually lasting for minutes.

The rub is that migraine *often* causes TIA-*like* symptoms without also causing major headache that might favor its recognition. Consequently, neurological symptoms of migraine sometimes are misinterpreted as TIAs caused by blood clots, and treatment thus is misdirected, sometimes dangerously. In part it happens because—understandably—doctors tend to "err on the side of caution." But it also reflects inadequate awareness of the full spectrum of migraine. And the so-called side of caution, when it's the wrong side that leads to unnecessary, dangerous treatment, is *not* the safe side.

How Tests Can Mislead

I HAVE SEEN numerous patients with fleeting neurological symptoms such as transient visual loss or numbness—due to migraine—who as a result of these symptoms have undergone carotid artery surgery or been placed on long-term anticoagulation (blood-thinning medication) because of misdiagnosis that their symptoms were due to blood clots from a carotid artery or the heart. This scenario is a good example of how tests can do more harm than good.

Sometimes clinical judgment by an astute doctor is sufficient to identify, accurately and confidently, that migraine is the source of TIA-like episodes. If, however, tests of the carotid arteries and heart are obtained, there may be positive findings that are *asymptomatic* and *inconsequential* but nonetheless command attention. Test findings may outweigh clinical judgment, leading away from diagnosis and treat-

"But they told me to drink red wine!"

MIRANDA'S STORY

When Miranda started having 20-minute episodes of left visual loss at age 75, her doctors figured it was some sort of problem with blood clots and treated her with a blood thinner even though all her tests in this area were normal. The episodes continued, and by the time I saw her, Miranda was also having "dull headaches" daily. Sensing migraine, I had Miranda follow the diet. (Ironically, one of her doctors had told her to drink two glasses of red wine each night to unclog her blood vessels!)

After two months on the diet, Miranda was symptom-free: no spells of visual loss, and no headaches. She then began to liberalize the diet and had minor visual episodes in response to Canadian bacon, cheese, hot dogs and lemonade, as well as with intense stress. Overall, she felt "much better" and found the dietary limitations to be quite tolerable. ◆

ment of the true problem—migraine—and toward unnecessary carotid artery surgery or anticoagulation.

I'm not saying that tests aren't at times reasonable or even essential, sometimes just to sort out problems that ultimately turn out to be due to migraine. Rather, I'm saying that the correct diagnosis and treatment of migraine—or of any problem with which migraine might be confused—depends in the end on wise clinical judgment. In some cases, tests can distort and distract, rather than focus, a doctor's diagnostic vision.

BEYOND MIGRAINE

CHAPTER NINE

When Treatment Fails

Conventional headache diagnosis and treatment routinely lead to failure. Headaches are mislabeled, rebound is ignored, avoidable triggers are not eliminated and preventive medications aren't used effectively. With *proper* diagnosis and treatment of migraine, headache control can almost always be achieved. *Almost* always. Why does even optimal treatment—the 1-2-3 Program—sometimes fail?

Recognizing and Treating Depression

SOMETIMES TREATMENT FAILS because of concurrent, untreated depression. Depression and migraine trigger and reinforce each other in a vicious cycle and should be treated in concert. A tricyclic antidepressant, such as nortriptyline, may serve both purposes. On the other hand, certain treatments for one of these problems can make the other one worse.

Prescribing selective serotonin reuptake inhibitors such as fluoxetine (Prozac) for depression can provoke headaches in some people, and beta blockers for migraine prevention can aggravate depression.

Depression not only triggers migraine but interferes with its treatment. Depression saps your motivation, drains your energy and dims your hope, all of which you need if you're going to take the necessary steps to control your headaches. A headache sufferer with depression is less likely to do the right things.

To make matters worse, depression often goes unrecognized or is denied by those in its grip for a number of reasons, beginning with loss of insight—an integral defect of depression. People who are depressed are often the last to acknowledge it, despite the torrents of tears they shed just from reading Hallmark cards or watching Kodak ads. In addition, when you're depressed, you may argue that you're *not* depressed because you don't *feel* sad or because you have no reason to be depressed.

Depression need not cause sadness. Its primary symptoms may be fatigue, insomnia and forgetfulness, without feeling blue. And depression occurs routinely *without* a clear reason, presumably on a biochemical basis. *The message is:* When migraine treatment fails, consider—and reconsider—the possibility that depression is complicating things, and consider treating that possibility.

Hidden Agendas

ANOTHER COMMON REASON that proper treatment fails is some hidden agenda that either interferes with your compliance with treatment, blocks your favorable response to treatment, inhibits your willingness to report favorable treatment response, or all of the above. Personal injury and disability claims dependent on headache complaints are prime examples. If you're suing someone for being negligent and caus-

The Trap of Disability Status

Think about it. If you were excused from work but still received a paycheck as long as you complained of headaches, wouldn't you be tempted to keep on complaining? Don't you think this might interfere not only with your motivation to respond to treatment, but also with your willingness to report favorable response?

The two essential goals of treating chronic headaches are to control your headaches and to maximize your functional status, a more objective measure comprising your activities, including work. These goals should be sought in concert and are mutually reinforcing. It makes no sense for a doctor to undermine the second goal by supporting long-term disability claims based on headache complaints. Yet it happens often.

Why? First, endorsing disability claims for headaches is the path of least resistance. The patient who walks out of a doctor's office with a signed disability form is grateful and content, in contrast to the one who departs angrily with an unsigned form. Second, signing disability forms may be an exercise of power that gratifies some doctors. Third, helping a "failed" headache patient obtain long-term disability also may benefit the doctor. When a patient is certified as "disabled," treatment failure is *legitimized* and the doctor is unburdened of any potential responsibility.

If you've sought long-term disability status because of headaches, you might protest that I must not understand the extent of your suffering. You would be wrong. I not only understand your suffering, I also know that you've never been treated properly.

Disability claims are a lot like rebound. You may say, *I can't give up my quick fixes until my headaches are under control!* I say, *Your headaches never will be under control until you give up your quick fixes.* You say, *I can't go back to work until my headaches are under control!* I say, *Your headaches never will be under control until you give up your disability claim and go back to work.* Like rebound, disability is a trap: it guarantees that you'll be complaining of headache until you choose to set yourself free. ◆

A Question

How do I reconcile my comments about psychological and emotional issues impeding treatment response with my criticism of doctors who assume that headache sufferers complain for psychological and emotional reasons?

In my experience, very few headache sufferers fail *proper* treatment as a result of psychological and emotional issues, unlike the many patients judged to be failures after not responding to conventional headache (mis)diagnosis and (mis)-treatment. Moreover, rather than deeming chronic headache complaints "psychosomatic" and attributing them to character deficiencies, I believe that most such complaints have a physical basis: migraine. It's just that psychological and emotional issues can block some people from doing the right things to control migraine or can amplify their complaints. ◆

ing you injury, and if headaches are a major aspect of damages or grounds for a disability claim, you have potentially powerful motivation (whether or not you're aware of it and no matter how much you deny it) not to comply with or respond well to treatment. Or at least to report poor response.

I'll tell you this: When I first see a headache patient, I almost invariably feel optimistic about that patient's eventual outcome, and it turns out that I'm almost always right. But I have to admit that I've learned to be less optimistic, and am more likely to be ultimately disappointed, when the patient is entrenched in or seeking disability status, or pursuing a lawsuit, based on headaches. These are far and away the biggest reasons for treatment failure in my own hands.

Hidden agendas can be more subtle, as when we reap rewards from being in the sick role. When we're sick, others give us their attention, concern, affection, sympathy, help, forgiveness and permission to be excused from work and other responsibilities. As a neurologist friend of mine has noted, we all like having our pillows fluffed.

Beneath the radar screen of our awareness, our subconscious may have some other hidden agenda that interferes with response to treatment. We all struggle with our identities. Being identified as a headache patient—

especially a *failed* headache patient—may actually be valuable to some people. At least it's *some* identity; it distinguishes you. Giving this up leaves a vacuum, and filling the void may not be so easy.

Sometimes It's Hard to Let Go

LETTING GO OF HEADACHES can be tricky for other reasons. Chronic headache sufferers know all too well that family and friends sometimes wonder whether their headaches are "real." Controlling your headaches, especially if accomplished fairly simply with proper preventive treatment, may make you worry, and others wonder, whether the whole problem *was* "just in your head." It's not, but you may worry anyway— at least subconsciously—enough to hold you back from letting go of your headaches.

Also holding you back may be the implications of this question: *You mean I've suffered needlessly with headaches all these years?* The anger, regret and sorrow stirred up by this question can be too much to bear. You turn away, in denial of any prospect of a new life. Or, you may be too mired in guilt, believing that you deserve your headaches, or just too weary and hopeless to conceive that renewing the effort to control your headaches is worthwhile, so you don't try hard enough.

Counseling may be helpful in understanding and overcoming resistance to treatment success, but be careful. Counselors, in the mistaken belief that chronic headaches are caused by muscle tension secondary to stress and anxiety, often emphasize relaxation techniques rather than help you confront difficult psychological and emotional issues that keep you from controlling your headaches. Sometimes, counseling of headache sufferers is misdirected toward helping people to cope with rather than *control* their headaches. The helping-you-cope approach is based on the premise that you're stuck with your headaches. You're not.

CHAPTER TEN

When It's Not Migraine

A side from migraine, the other noteworthy primary headache disorder—that is, a headache problem that has a life of its own as opposed to one that is secondary to some underlying disease—is *cluster headache*. Unlike migraine, which is universal (though highly variable among us), cluster headache is a distinctive problem that afflicts a relatively small number of people, mostly men. Later in this chapter we'll consider when to look for trouble: when is a head CT or MRI scan a good idea (and when isn't it) to look for something other than migraine or cluster?

Cluster Headache

LIKE MIGRAINE, cluster headache involves a mechanism that is based in the brain and generates swelling and inflammation of blood vessels around the head, but certain features set it apart. "Cluster" refers to its typical temporal pattern: intervals lasting weeks to months, at certain seasons of the year, interspersed with longer headache-free intervals. During a headache interval, headaches usually occur one to several times daily, lasting about one-half to one hour. Often these headaches begin in sleep, specifically in rapid eye movement (REM, or dream) sleep, but they may appear during wakefulness as well, sometimes like clockwork.

The pain of cluster headache is excruciating and localized around one eye, always on the same side within a cluster interval and usually on the same side from one interval to the next. Commonly there is associated redness and tearing of the eye, and sometimes drooping of the eyelid and reduced size of the pupil. The nose and sinuses become congested on the painful side. In the midst of a cluster headache, the sufferer is likely to be restless and agitated—not quiet and withdrawn, as during severe migraine. Suicidal thoughts are common. Descriptions of cluster headache sound like something from hell.

Symptoms associated with full-blown migraine, such as vomiting and visual disturbances, are absent in cluster headache. Alcohol is a potent and immediate trigger of cluster headache during a cluster interval (though not during headache-free intervals), but other migraine dietary triggers don't per-

"Secondary" Headaches

This book is *not* about the many, many diseases, including serious conditions such as tumors, infection or bleeding involving the brain, that *can* cause headache but, in the universe of headaches, are relatively rare. *Secondary* headaches— those that arise from some underlying disease—tend to have distinguishing features that doctors are trained to recognize. The presumption of this book is that you and your doctor have excluded any such problem and that you have a *primary* headache disorder: migraine (or, less likely, cluster). ◆

tain to cluster. Smoking tobacco, which doesn't seem to be an important trigger of migraine, may contribute to cluster headache.

As with migraine, there are two forms of treatment for cluster headache: acute and preventive. Also as with migraine, preventive treatment is best. Cluster intervals usually begin gradually, with several or more days of worsening headaches prior to reaching full force. At the first sign, a preventive medication is initiated (see Table 10, page 189). Ideally, favorable experience with a preventive medication during a prior cluster interval dictates its repeated use and optimal dosage. Otherwise, one medication is chosen from the list, and you increase the dosage rapidly over one to two weeks—more aggressively than in preventive

---

"I lost three teeth for nothing!"

LEE'S STORY

To me, the diagnosis of cluster headache in Lee couldn't have been more obvious: a textbook story of indescribably severe pain around his right eye, with redness and tearing, lasting up to an hour, waking him every night, occurring every fall for a few months and then disappearing for a year. Yet he'd been misdiagnosed for years with allergies, sinus infection, dental problems (leading to three unnecessary tooth extractions!) and "stress." When headaches struck, he thought about killing himself.

It was such a pity, because he was so easy to treat: verapamil helped a lot, and the addition of divalproex worked perfectly. Now he cycles onto these medications whenever his cluster headaches heat up, and comes off them when the headaches cool down. Lee's very glad to be alive. ◆

Preventive Medication for Cluster Headache

	INITIAL DOSAGE	MAXIMAL DOSAGE OR SERUM LEVEL
CALCIUM CHANNEL BLOCKERS Verapamil or diltiazem	120 mg twice daily	240 to 480 mg twice daily
DIVALPROEX SODIUM	250 mg twice daily (or, in extended-release form, 500 mg at bedtime)	1,000 mg twice daily or level greater than 200 mcg/ml
PREDNISONE	60 to 80 mg daily, then taper	——
METHYSERGIDE	2 mg twice daily	4 mg three times daily
LITHIUM CARBONATE	300 mg twice daily	600 to 900 mg twice daily, or level greater than 1.5 mEq/l

Table 10

medication trials for migraine. (Prednisone is an exception: you start it at high dosage and then taper it.)

If it works satisfactorily, you continue the preventive medication for the anticipated duration of the cluster interval and then taper it, in the hope that the problem will have subsided. If withdrawal of preventive medication leads to recurrent headaches, you reinstitute the drug, and you can attempt to withdraw it again a few weeks or more later. If the chosen medication doesn't work satisfactorily after at least one week at maximal dosage, you substitute the next option in its place (if the first option was unhelpful) or add the next option to the mix (if the first option is partially beneficial).

You'll notice that the list of medications to control cluster headaches is similar—but not identical—to that for migraine. Tricyclic antidepressants and beta blockers, useful for migraine, aren't helpful for cluster headache. Lithium doesn't help migraine but is effective in a cluster headache, especially in a chronic form in which there are no headache-free intervals.

The best acute treatments for cluster headache are either inhalation of 100 percent oxygen or injection of sumatriptan. Oral triptans and opioids work too slowly to be very useful for individual cluster headaches, which are by nature relatively short-lived.

When to Look for Trouble

THE DIAGNOSIS AND TREATMENT of headaches secondary to tumors, infection or bleeding involving the brain is beyond the scope of this book, except for one issue: when is a head CT or MRI scan in order? In other words, when is it time to look for trouble?

Most chronic headache sufferers do not need scans for diagnosis. Their headaches are due to migraine (or infrequently, cluster), which is identified by history and can't be diagnosed by a scan. When something else more serious is causing headaches—something you would want to know about and act upon—it tends to let you know. In such cases, red flags are usually visible to your doctor, who is trained to recognize them.

For instance, the explosive onset of a uniquely severe headache may suggest intracranial hemorrhage and warrant scanning. Headaches associated with new-onset seizures may suggest a brain tumor. Relentlessly progressive headaches may spell trouble. Abnormal findings on neurological examination—findings that can't otherwise be explained reasonably—may be reason to consider a scan. Or, failure to respond to proper treatment (the 1-2-3 Program) for presumed migraine might justify a scan.

Odds are good that even when a dramatic headache (or a substantial change in headaches or some other symptom) prompts a scan, it will be normal. Up to a point, that's as it should be. If *every* scan of a headache patient were abnormal, revealing a brain tumor or ruptured aneurysm or some other serious cause of headache, this would suggest that not enough scans were being done and that such problems were being missed.

Sometimes scans aren't performed when they should be, but from my perspective of seeing thousands of chronic headache patients, the more common problem is not too *few* scans: it's too *many*. There's a balance between not overlooking serious problems and not overdoing scans, and the balance is out of whack. Partly it's because of the shortcomings of conventional headache wisdom, which breeds insecurity in doctors who are confronted with headache complaints they can't readily pigeonhole or resolve. And partly it's fear of lawsuits.

Too often, scans are intended not so much for diagnosis as for treatment: either treatment of the patient's anxiety about a possible brain tumor, aneurysm, stroke or whatever, or treatment of the doctor's concern about missing a diagnosis—however unlikely—and facing a lawsuit. Reassurance by a normal scan is potentially therapeutic for both patient and doctor.

But there's a catch. Without enough red flags to justify it, a scan "just to be on the safe side" amounts to looking for trouble without justification—and that often backfires. The likelihood of a scan showing the cause of headaches in a patient with chronic headaches and an unremarkable neurological examination—with no red flags—is minuscule. A much greater likelihood is that the scan will show *something*—but something that has *nothing* to do with the symptoms at hand. At best, this *increases* anxiety. At worst it pushes the patient and doctor down an irresistible but ultimately dangerous path that leads to more unnecessary tests, unnecessary treatment and unnecessary trouble.

I have seen this scenario unfold time and again. A scan (or some other test) that didn't need to be done shows an incidental finding, but its incidental nature may not be appreciated. Indeed, the undeniability

"The verdict was hydrocephalus"

FRANK'S AND JANET'S STORIES

I met Frank too late to help him avoid brain surgery. His chronic headaches had prompted an MRI scan that revealed a cyst thought to be blocking spinal fluid flow out of his brain and thereby causing hydrocephalus. When I did meet him, a year after surgery to drain the cyst and decompress his brain had failed to relieve his headaches, I reviewed the films and it was apparent that these findings were of no consequence and should have gone untouched. His headaches stemmed from migraine, in this case complicated by rebound from Fioricet. He stopped it (Step 1), followed the diet (Step 2) and adjusted his preventive medications (Step 3). His subsequent self-reports over a four-year period improved from "much better" to "great."

Think Frank's story is unique? Unfortunately, it's not. Ten years ago, Janet came to me with an almost identical story. She'd had chronic headaches due to migraine (plus rebound) since she was a teenager, but in her mid-thirties a CT scan showed hydrocephalus and a shunt was placed to siphon off fluid. Her headaches persisted because hydrocephalus wasn't the problem.

For six months after we first met, Janet did well by addressing migraine and rebound, but she got sidetracked. Sadly, of the 70 shunt operations she's undergone to deal with infections and presumed malfunctions, 40 of them took place during the 10 years since I last saw her. And frighteningly, I suspect that many of those procedures were actually performed in response to unrecognized flare-ups of migraine fueled by rebound from eight or more Excedrin and several Tylox daily. Now, having initially benefited from the 1-2-3 Program, Janet has come back to carry it through. ◆

of the finding (you can see it with your own eyes!) and the report of the finding—in black and white—overwhelm clinical judgment. Thus headaches come to be mistakenly attributed to asymptomatic structural abnormalities in the sinuses, or simple cysts or small benign tumors of no consequence within the skull, or a vascular malformation (a usually innocent tangle of blood vessels), or other longstanding *non*issues such as an Arnold-Chiari malformation or compensated hydrocephalus (enlargement of the fluid-filled cavities in the brain, but without persistently increased pressure in them). In some cases, needless treatment is undertaken and surgery may be performed.

Even when the scan finding doesn't lead to treatment such as surgery, the patient nonetheless is left to live with uncertainty. *Is this the cause of my headaches . . . or not? Will it eventually have to be treated? What will happen if it isn't!*

A variation on this theme is the unnecessary MRI scan showing small, bright spots in the brain that are overinterpreted as strokes or as lesions of multiple sclerosis. Such spots are common, nonspecific and usually insignificant—and may be associated with migraine. But because similar findings *can* be seen with strokes or multiple sclerosis,

Less Is More

Maybe it's no secret that, as a general rule, the best doctors prescribe the least medication. But the best doctors also order the fewest tests—only those that are *truly necessary*. At least, it sure looks that way from where I stand.

Unfortunately, the right combination of wisdom, confidence and courage (needed to resist the wrongheaded forces that urge more and more testing) seems in short supply. ◆

these diagnoses are sometimes mentioned in scan reports. Especially when you have neurological symptoms from unrecognized migraine, there is the risk that a misdiagnosis such as stroke or multiple sclerosis will stick. The potential consequences of such misdiagnoses are grave: not only anxiety and fear, but further (and increasingly dangerous) tests and treatments.

Scans are double-edged swords that should be wielded wisely. Sometimes you create trouble by looking for it. A principle of medicine is: *First, do no harm.* In headache patients without clear-cut red flags, scans do more harm than good. Therefore: *First, do no scan.* Unless, of course, there's a good reason—legitimate diagnostic concern—and not just a need for reassurance based on ignorance of the spectrum of migraine and insecurity bred by fear of lawsuits.

A Dialogue

PART OF BEING A GOOD DOCTOR lies in understanding what's on your patients' minds—their fears and confusion, their skepticism and stubbornness (not to mention their hopes and dreams). And no doctor can do that without listening carefully to what patients are saying. I'd like to think that I've become a good doctor to my headache patients by listening. Here's a sampling of what I hear most frequently—and of what I say in return.

How do I know I don't have a brain tumor?

In 20 years of practicing neurology, I've seen my share of people with brain tumors, but I have yet to see one who just had headaches. Brain tumors usually cause seizures, mental changes such as confusion, or some other neurological problem—and may produce headaches but rarely in isolation.

But shouldn't I have a head scan, just to be sure?

Maybe . . . but probably not. Your doctor should be able to recognize the red flags in your history or your examination that might justify risking the downsides of scanning: principally, that some incidental finding will open not a can but a *big barrel* of worms.

What do you mean, "red flags"?

> For example, if you have the sudden onset of the worst headache of your life or your headaches are relentlessly progressive. Or, obviously, if you have a new onset of seizures or some other worrisome neurological problem along with your headaches.

Could the sudden, sharp pains in my head mean that I've developed an aneurysm?

> It's ironic that these brief but intense pains that terrify you are, to a knowledgeable doctor, the *least* concerning of all headache descriptions, because they're the least likely to arise from anything serious, or anything at all other than migraine.

What does an aneurysm feel like?

> Generally, there's no feeling at all . . . unless it ruptures. In that case, you're likely to suddenly have a uniquely severe headache that won't quit.

Then shouldn't I have a scan to make sure I don't have an aneurysm before that happens to me?

> No, that's a bad idea.

Why?

> Because you might actually find one!

WHAT?

> Suppose you turn out to have an unruptured aneurysm. Consider two possible scenarios: (1) the aneurysm never would have ruptured, but you undergo surgery (in which it's clipped) and you suffer a serious complication, or (2) the aneurysm would have ruptured, but thankfully you have successful, uncomplicated sur-

gery before that happens. Which do you think is vastly more likely? (Hint: it's not the latter.) Now consider a third scenario: you don't have surgery, the aneurysm never ruptures, but you live the rest of your life fearing that it will pop at any moment if you strain too much or get really upset or . . .

Okay, but if I don't have a brain tumor or an aneurysm, why are my headaches getting worse?

Hold on: that *might* be a red flag that merits investigation. But assuming that you don't have something else going on, your increased headaches reflect increased migraine activity—which means that your threshold has dropped, or (more likely) your trigger level has risen, or (least likely) both.

But nothing's changed as far as I can tell, except that my headaches are worse.

Maybe nothing's changed, or maybe something *has* changed and you just don't get it or you're denying it. For instance, it seems to me that people often deny that they're under unusual stress—and thereby having more headaches—because denial helps them cope with whatever is stressing them out. Yet they deny the fact that they're in denial.

No, no, I'm not under more stress.

Okay, then. For whatever unknown reason, the balance between your threshold and your trigger level has tipped unfavorably. The important thing is, by using the 1-2-3 Program you can restore the balance in your favor.

My headaches aren't necessarily worse—they're just different. Why?

It's the nature of migraine to cause different forms of head (and face and neck) discomfort at different times. Sometimes these different headaches commingle, and sometimes they change from one to another as you go through life.

Do you mean to say that virtually every kind of headache is generated by migraine?

Yes. And everyone has it.

Well, what is a migraine, anyway?

Don't think of *a* migraine. Think of *migraine*: the mechanism. Don't think of migraine as any particular type of headache; think of it as a mechanism that can generate all types of headaches and plenty of other symptoms if your trigger level exceeds your threshold and depending on how much.

Why do I get more headaches than most people?

That's easy: mainly because your migraine threshold is lower than most people's, and maybe partly because your trigger level is relatively higher.

Can I thank my parents for my low threshold?

Yes.

But their headaches are nowhere near as bad as mine. They don't have migraine.

They do. We all do, to varying degrees. Migraine doesn't "breed true." You can be worse off—or better off—than your parents. Also, family members may be relatively silent sufferers. Or they may not complain of "migraine," just of "sinus" or some other misdiagnosis of migraine.

So are my children doomed to suffer from headaches?

I wouldn't look at it that way. It's true that their likelihood of having headache problems is higher if you're a headache sufferer. But even if they're not lucky enough to escape your genetic influence, they—like all people who get headaches—can control their tendency with the 1-2-3 Program.

Will my headaches get better when I get older?

That's the general trend, especially in postmenopausal women who don't take any form of hormone replacement. But there are a fair number of exceptions to the rule . . . even some folks who experience their first headaches when they reach their sixties or seventies.

Why am I so tired? Is it migraine?

Migraine wears you down. Headaches, neck stiffness, sinus congestion, dizziness and the many other symptoms of migraine are a heavy burden to bear. Also, medications that you take to treat these symptoms may be making you tired. Plus, if your sleep is disrupted by migraine, or you become worried or depressed, these factors take a further toll on your energy.

And maybe migraine directly produces fatigue as a physical consequence of its mechanism unfolding. I don't know exactly how this would happen, but there sure are a lot of people suffering from chronic headaches and other symptoms of migraine who also feel unduly fatigued, suggesting that both arise from common ground.

It's striking how much more energetic people feel once they've gained control of their headaches.

I hurt all over! Is that migraine?

The primary territory of migraine is in and around your head, face and neck, including your "shoulders" (trapezius muscle regions) and shoulder blades (upper back), but no shortage of my patients initially complain of low back pain as well. I tell them I can't promise that this will resolve along with their more straightforward discomfort (after all, chronic low back pain is very common and has many causes, unrelated to migraine), but it often *does* improve as migraine is controlled.

Why?

I'm not sure. I don't believe that migraine *directly* produces low back pain, and I don't understand why some people with chronic low back pain feel better when migraine is treated properly; it's just that some do. Maybe they would have improved anyway.

What about pain elsewhere?

Occasionally, migraine will cause arm or leg discomfort (usually vague aching, sometimes associated with feelings of heaviness, or numbness and tingling) and perhaps also abdominal pain (so-called abdominal migraine). Incidentally, quite a few headache patients I see have been previously labeled with fibromyalgia or myofascial pain syndrome, because of their widespread pain complaints. Apart from the role that depression and other psychological and emotional influences can play in making someone hurt all over, it's been

my experience that most of these individuals suffer from migraine
. . . and feel better all over when they follow the 1-2-3 Program.

How do I know I'm not crazy? Other people seem to think I must be
if I have a headache every day.

You may be crazy in other respects, but you're not imagining that
your head hurts every day, due to daily activation of migraine, or
that the degree of pain correlates with your stress level (in combination with a lot of other triggers.) And you can prove you're *not* all
that crazy using the 1-2-3 Program to control your headaches.

Why do I wake up virtually every morning with a headache?

This may be a clue to rebound, if you're withdrawing from quick
fixes overnight. Or you may be withdrawing from dietary caffeine.
These explanations are especially likely if you feel somewhat better
in the morning after you feed your quick-fix habit or take care of
your coffee jones.

Occasionally, sleep apnea (breathing pauses during sleep)
contributes to morning headaches, maybe by acting as a migraine
trigger. But many people wake up every morning with headaches
simply because their trigger levels are *constantly* above their thresholds—and especially if their daily migraine rhythm consists of a
natural, preprogrammed rise in trigger level at that time. Just don't
assume you wake up with headaches because you "slept wrong."

But my headaches seem to be related to how I move my head and neck.

I explain this apparent relationship in Chapter Seven. The bottom line is, the problem is usually migraine, and the solution to migraine is the 1-2-3 Program.

Why does the weather give me headaches?

Various aspects of weather, especially barometric pressure changes (as when storms approach), temperature changes or extremes (for some people it's heat, for others cold, and for still others a change either way), high humidity and bright sunlight (or glare), feed into your migraine control center and stack on top of other triggers until your trigger level exceeds your threshold.

You mean it's not my sinuses?

Right! Unless you're referring to *migraine* affecting your sinuses by causing blood vessels within them to become swollen and in-flamed, thereby producing congestion and so-called sinus headache. But if you think that storms somehow trigger your headaches on an *allergic* basis, you're all wet. Let me ask *you* a question: Why would that be? The answer is: It wouldn't . . . it isn't . . . it doesn't make any sense. Yet many people imagine that their weather-related headaches somehow reflect allergies, as part of the perva-sive mythology under which the truth of migraine lies buried.

But my headaches are worse in the spring and fall. Isn't that because of allergies?

Are you really *sure* you're substantially, consistently worse at those times? I ask that because my experience has been that many of my new patients initially make this claim, but the more I delve into their history, the clearer it becomes that their headaches are year-round—not limited to times of high pollen counts. If you really think about it, maybe this applies to you, too.

And even if you're right about your headaches being *exclusively* seasonal (which would make you relatively rare in my experience), and even if the seasonal connection is allergic rather than something else, I still maintain that the problem-causing mechanism is migraine, with allergic activity no more than a triggering influence, and that a migraine-preventive approach—the 1-2-3 Program—is the solution.

Sometimes I get a headache when I exercise. What should I do?
Keep exercising.

And suffer headaches?
No. You should exercise *and* follow the 1-2-3 Program to control your headaches. That way you'll be able to tolerate whatever triggering effect exercise might have, without getting headaches. And in the long run, regular exercise can actually play a role in preventing your headaches—not to mention helping you feel better, sleep better, lose weight, look better and be healthier.

How long will it take me to get over rebound when I stop taking my Excedrin?
Up to a few weeks. (This is also true of similar quick fixes such as Fioriet and Imitrex.) At first you may find it difficult not having a crutch to lean on. And there's about a fifty-fifty chance that

you'll actually have increased headaches for up to a few weeks as a result of withdrawal. But any temporary suffering is a whole lot less than the future suffering you're guaranteed if you continue to rebound.

It's been a week since I stopped taking my quick-fix medications, and my headaches are worse. What can I take for the pain?

Only plain acetaminophen or aspirin (*without caffeine*), or an anti-inflammatory medication such as ibuprofen or naproxen.

But I've tried them, and they don't work. What else can I take?

For pain, that's it for now. If you take a rebound-causing quick fix, you'll backstep and never get control over your headaches.

What about for nausea and vomiting?

An antiemetic (see Table 3, page 41) won't cause rebound, and its sedating effect might not be a bad thing if you're already bed-bound.

How often can I take a triptan?

If you're in a rebound situation related to *any* rebound-causing quick fix, not just a triptan, the answer is: *Not at all.* At least not until you've controlled your headaches satisfactorily for at least four months. If you're *not* rebounding, you may take a triptan up to a maximum of two days per month without risking rebound.

What can I take if I have a cold?

Stay away from decongestants if possible, because they can cause rebound headaches. It's okay to take acetaminophen or aspirin (*without caffeine*), or ibuprofen or naproxen. Antihistamines are also okay, as are expectorants (such as guaifenesin) and cough sup-

pressants (dextromethorphan, codeine), as long as they're not combined with a decongestant. Antibiotics are fine as well.

Of all the potential dietary triggers, what are the real biggies?

As a general rule: caffeine, caffeine and caffeine . . . plus chocolate,
MSG, nitrite-processed meats, aged cheeses, nuts (and peanut butter) and alcohol (maybe just certain types, like red wine). Also, for
many people, yogurt, citrus (including pineapples), bananas, onions
and aspartame (NutraSweet).

*That's not so bad. You mean I can put a major dent in my trigger level
and maybe get it below my threshold just by avoiding the items you
mentioned?*

Major dent, yes; below threshold, don't count on it. You'd be wiser
to avoid all the dietary items discussed as triggers in Chapter
Four, at least in the beginning. Then, once you've controlled
your headaches, you can better afford to experiment.

*After I've controlled my headaches, how long do I have to wait before I
can start experimenting with the foods you want me to avoid?*

Not until you've had at least *four months* of satisfactory headache
control. See Chapter Four to find the best ways to reintroduce foods
to your diet, and consult the Dietary Tips in the Appendix.

*Since I have headaches with my periods, wouldn't it be a good idea for
me to take birth-control pills?*

No. That would be throwing fuel on the fire—at least where most
women are concerned. Yes, some cases have proved the exception,
but these are relatively few in my experience.

I've been taking Prozac (or Paxil, Zoloft, Effexor or Wellbutrin . . .) for depression, and I swear my headaches have gotten worse. When I told my doctor, he said no way. I think he just thought I was even crazier.

How crazy you are may still be a legitimate matter of debate, but the headache-stimulating effect of these drugs—in some people, at least—is not debatable. It's not your imagination, it's for real.

You recommend adjusting treatment for depression in order to avoid the headache-stimulating potential of certain antidepressant medications and instead benefit from the migraine-preventive effect of another type. But my doctor doesn't want to change my antidepressant medication. What should I do?

Make sure your doctor understands what's at stake. Does he or she know how much you suffer from headaches? Or that the underlying mechanism, migraine, can be aggravated by some antidepressants and suppressed by others? Get the issues out in the open.

Maybe your doctor's right and your treatment for depression shouldn't be modified, at least for the time being. If so, this can be revisited down the road, depending in part on how you respond to the other changes you can make using the 1-2-3 Program.

My blood pressure is low to begin with. What will happen if I take a blood pressure medicine to help prevent my headaches?

Most likely, nothing, except that it will help prevent your headaches. Don't worry that it will lower your blood pressure further. As a rule, blood pressure medicine mainly lowers *high* blood pressure. In fact, I would suggest that you not even check to see if it lowers your blood pressure further. If it lowered it too much, you'd know, because you'd feel lightheaded whenever you stand up. Otherwise, even if your blood pressure is somewhat lower, it doesn't matter.

But isn't low blood pressure why I feel tired all the time? And won't the blood pressure medicine make me feel even more tired?

It's a misconception that people feel tired all the time because of low blood pressure. There are lots of reasons for feeling tired, but that's not one of them. And while it's true that beta blockers sometimes cause fatigue, this effect is not directly related to lowering of blood pressure; it has to do with the way these blood pressure medicines block adrenaline. Other blood pressure medicines that lower blood pressure just as much but don't block adrenaline will not cause fatigue.

I'm not depressed, and I feel reluctant about taking an antidepressant medication to prevent migraine.

The effect of tricyclic antidepressants in preventing migraine is independent of their antidepressant action; you don't have to be depressed to benefit. But an individual who *is* depressed can kill two birds with one stone (and also sleep better, without sleeping pills).

I've read the pamphlet that comes with one of the medications you recommend for migraine prevention, and it says that one of the side effects is headaches! Should I take it?

The proliferation of lists warning about potential side effects of medications is characteristic of the butt-covering mentality that pervades our society. Having gotten that off my chest, I agree that you should know about reasonably possible side effects of any medication you take. But headaches are *not* a likely reaction to any of the migraine-preventive options discussed in Chapter Five.

I'm still afraid my headaches might get worse. What should I do?
You should be careful: not that your headaches might get worse, but that you will talk yourself into experiencing side effects that wouldn't have occurred if you'd just calmed down and assumed a more positive mindset. If you *do* script your own treatment failure, one medication after the next, pretty soon you'll be out of options, including a number that would have helped you if you'd only given them a chance.

Isn't antiseizure medication dangerous? Why should I take it for migraine prevention?
Divalproex, the antiseizure medication that is effective for migraine prevention, is not dangerous—at least no more so than most medications. The potential side effects that are reasonable possibilities are nuisance issues, not life-threatening problems. Anyone who overblows this issue is guilty of butt-covering at the expense of your potential benefit from divalproex.

If I take preventive medication, will I need a lot of blood tests?
No. Only divalproex requires a few blood tests, and that's only temporarily at the beginning of treatment.

The migraine-preventive medication I tried made me constipated. What should I do?

Maybe you should try it again, using a lower dosage (at least initially) and letting your body adjust to the medication. If you're patient, you'll often find that initial side effects fade over time.

Constipation can be further managed by drinking lots of fluids (especially water), staying physically active (ideally by exercising regularly) and bulking up on fiber. Fiber can be obtained by dietary means, such as fruits (strawberries, apples) and cereals (bran especially), or with a supplement (ask your pharmacist). If you use prunes, watch out for those preserved with sulfites: a trigger.

I'm gaining weight from my preventive medication. What should I do?

Start with understanding that although this problem *may* be due to the medication (that is, tricyclic antidepressants, divalproex and cyproheptadine can all stimulate your appetite and encourage you to eat more), the potential solution is in *your* hands: restricting caloric intake (watching what you eat) and increasing caloric expenditure (exercising). Hopefully you can exert the necessary dietary control and physical effort to overcome any heightened hunger you may experience. If not, you have to decide if the extra poundage is worth the additional headache control that the medication provides. If you decide it's not, you can try a different preventive medication, keeping in mind that the different medications that can lead to weight gain are just that—*different.* And while one may affect you that way, another may not.

I'm taking the tricyclic amitriptyline for headache prevention, but it's not helping and I can't increase the dosage because it makes me sleepy.

Ask your doctor about switching to nortriptyline, which works every bit as well but is less sedating. Try taking it earlier in the evening to better avoid sedation first thing in the morning. And go up with the dosage by *small* steps, using combinations of 10 and 25 mg capsules to achieve 5 or 10 mg dosage increments.

After a few days of taking a preventive medication, I got a headache and felt really dizzy. I don't want to try that medication again.

I can tell you from experience that it's more likely your headache and dizziness stemmed from migraine than from the medication. This happens all the time, and the solution is to *increase* the medication—not to stop it—and to take the other right steps to control migraine.

I really don't want to take a preventive medication every day.

I don't want you to, either. But sometimes it's the right thing to do. Are you sure you aren't already taking *something* for headaches—some kind of quick fix—almost every day? Or at least most days? Doesn't it make more sense to take a daily preventive medication that actually *works* rather than routinely suffering headaches and keeping your fingers crossed that you have a quick fix handy—and that it works? And if you're worried about side effects, you're wrong if you think the quick fixes you're using are any more benign than using a preventive medication.

Look, it boils down to this: You can't have everything you want. You can't eat whatever you want, and avoid taking preventive medication, *and* control your headaches. Nothing comes without a price, but preventive medication may be a real *bargain* when it comes to controlling your headaches.

How long will I need to keep taking a preventive medication?

However long you need to, which you can determine by trying to reduce or eliminate the medication whenever you choose and then seeing what happens. If you still need the medication, or at least a certain dosage of it, recurrent headaches or other migraine symptoms will let you know.

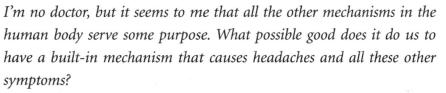

I'm no doctor, but it seems to me that all the other mechanisms in the human body serve some purpose. What possible good does it do us to have a built-in mechanism that causes headaches and all these other symptoms?

I can only guess why nature provided us with migraine—and why its level of activity is so high in so many people. Maybe migraine is the remnant of a primitive reflex that once led us to seek shelter in a cool, quiet, dark cave in response to potential threats. Or maybe it's a fluke: an evolutionary misstep that hasn't had enough reproductive *dis*advantage to lead it to a dead end.

On the other hand, perhaps migraine is an unavoidable by-product of the workings of the human brain—a necessary evil of our nature, if you will. This possibility is worth considering in light of what we know about seizures, which are also a natural by-product of the way our brains function. Every one of us has the potential to have a seizure. It's just a matter of sufficient provocation. Our brains function electrically, and accordingly a short circuit—a seizure—can be triggered in anybody. Some people are more apt to have seizures because they have lower thresholds. These individuals constitute the $^1/_2$ to 1 percent of the population with chronic seizure disorders. (An even greater percentage of people, maybe 5 percent, have had at least one seizure at some time in their lives.) The relationship between the level of seizure triggers and the seizure threshold determines the occurrence of a seizure in any of us.

Sound familiar? Although seizures and migraine are different phenomena, the parallels between them are many. Both are natural and universal: the potential to experience each is built into every one of us. Both have wide varieties of not only inputs (triggers) but also outputs (symptoms). Perhaps seizures and migraine have something else in common: maybe both are inescapable possibilities simply because of the way the human brain is wired to function.

Sometimes we see least clearly that which is too close for us to focus on: our nature. This much is clear: the mechanism of migraine is *physiological*—part of the way the human brain naturally functions. Migraine also can be *pathological*—like a disease—when its effects interfere with your quality of life. That's where the 1-2-3 Program comes in. Although migraine is natural, it is not necessary, thanks to proper treatment.

≋

Why didn't we know about all of this before?

Because generations of doctors have failed to question the mythology handed down about headaches. We've been told—and we've believed, without questioning—that migraine is one specific type of headache and anything different must be something else. For the most part, doctors have failed to question what they've been taught about headaches, despite overwhelming evidence—headache treatment failure, again and again—that the traditional "answers" are wrong. Moreover, most headache sufferers have simply accepted the standard answers offered by doctors while also accepting blame and bearing guilt for their headaches. Maybe we can learn something from the persistence of incorrect but unquestioned beliefs about headaches among so many people in so many different roles for so long—something about not only the practice of medicine but also human nature. *We should learn to question failure and not accept the excuses offered for it.*

There's an even darker side to the persistence of conventional wisdom—in truth, conventional *falsehoods*—about headaches. These falsehoods have become institutionalized. There are large and powerful industries that cater to headache sufferers misdiagnosed with tension headache, sinus headache and so many other misdiagnoses. For those individuals who are diagnosed correctly with migraine but who want a quick fix, there is no shortage of drug suppliers.

The financial investment in all of this, by many, is huge. If the realization that conventional wisdom is wrong were to catch on, the potential losses to those heavily invested in the status quo would be colossal. On the other hand, so would be the potential gains by the multitude of headache sufferers who finally would be correctly diagnosed with and *properly* treated for migraine.

Postscript

WHAT HAS ALWAYS MADE MIGRAINE DIFFICULT TO SEE CLEARLY is that the mechanism is triggered by so many different factors, all mixed together. And it expresses itself in so many different ways—even within an individual, let alone from person to person, varying over time—including all types of head, face and neck discomfort, with or without a wide array of non-headache symptoms. No wonder we've been confused. Rather than seeing the big picture, we've conjured links between specific inputs and outputs. Like the classic example of a group of sightless people feeling individual parts of an elephant and collectively describing a menagerie, we've failed to recognize the true nature of a single beast: migraine.

What ties together these multiple inputs and outputs is the solitary mechanism, migraine, that converts the complex mixture of triggers into these many symptoms. The beauty of it is, *you can control your symptoms with the 1-2-3 Program*: avoiding rebound, reducing your trigger exposure and, if necessary, blocking the mechanism using preventive medication. Understanding this is the key to controlling your headaches and other symptoms of migraine. *You now hold the key.* If you choose, you can unlock the door, walk through and be free.

"Forty years of headaches— and now I'm almost headache-free"

RUTH'S STORY

I t's Friday afternoon, November 30, 2001. In between seeing patients, I've been putting the finishing touches on this book. I thought I was just about done with it, but then Ruth came and I decided her story had to be told.

I initially evaluated Ruth four months ago: 40 years of headaches including "classic migraines" once a month; frequent "tension headaches" attributed to cervical spine disease and treated (unsuccessfully) with endless physical therapy; and "sinus-related" headaches for which she'd had years of allergy shots and three sinus surgeries without relief. Ruth was using Excedrin daily, and Tylenol Sinus and Fiorinal with Codeine each once or twice weekly. She was also on Premarin for estrogen replacement.

At that time I explained to Ruth what was going on—migraine, complicated by rebound—and what she needed to do about it: Step 1 (no more quick fixes) and Step 2 (substitution of estradiol for Premarin, and diet modification). She said it all made sense.

When Ruth returned today for her first follow-up, I asked her how she'd been doing with her headaches. Her response: "Much better." She'd done everything I suggested, and she was delighted with the outcome.

So, why did I feel compelled to share Ruth's story with you? Because it's exceptional? No, because it's routine. Every day, I hear stories like Ruth's—both the "before" and the "after." It's the "after" part that I really like. ◆

APPENDIX

Menus,
Recipes for Relief
and Dietary Tips

I don't want you to get the wrong idea: the items in the menus on the following pages are just *examples* of what you can eat. Unless, of course, you have other dietary concerns—reducing calories, lowering cholesterol, avoiding meat—that may preclude some of these items.

The good news is this: you could fill *shelves* of cookbooks with menus and recipes that are permitted within the confines of the migraine-preventive diet. You can adapt to the diet—even strictly—and still enjoy yourself, regardless of any additional dietary issues at hand. Be positive, be creative, and you can still eat, drink and be merry.

And remember, as time passes and you gain control over your headaches, you'll be able to liberalize the diet—if you wish—to at least some degree. As you read on, you'll see how well you can eat, starting with some menu ideas—they're just ideas—and then some recipes, followed by tips for both sticking with the diet and eventually relaxing it.

Menus

(Suggestions marked by diamonds include items featured in the recipe section.)

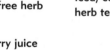

DAY 1

Breakfast

Bagel* with cream cheese

Pear

Caffeine-free herb tea

Cranberry juice

Lunch

♦ *Tuna salad* sandwich with lettuce and tomato

Grapes

Potato chips (salted but unflavored)

Caffeine-free cola (without aspartame)

Dinner

♦ Steak with *herb salsa*

String beans

Mashed potatoes

Apple pie with whipped cream

DAY 2

Breakfast

Scrambled eggs

Buttered toast

Kiwi

Caffeine-free herb tea

Mixed berry juice

Lunch

Roast beef sandwich

Celery sticks and olives

Iced, caffeine-free herb tea

Dinner

♦ *Crab cakes*

Corn

Baked potato with butter

♦ *Apricot cake*

Fruits & Juices *Help yourself to these fruits and their juices, but watch out for citrus blends! Raisins and other dried fruits naturally contain tyramine, which won't appear on the label; often they're also preserved with sulfites, which do appear on the label, so check before you buy. Since fruits in general accumulate tyramine as they ripen, choose young, fresh fruits whenever possible.*

APPLES	CANTALOUPE	HONEYDEW MELON	PEACHES
APRICOTS	CHERRIES	KIWI	PEARS
BLACKBERRIES	CRANBERRIES	MANGOES	STRAWBERRIES
BLUEBERRIES	GRAPES	NECTARINES	WATERMELON

---

*All yeast-risen baked goods, including the bagels, bread and muffins in these menus, should be one day or more out of the oven.

Breakfast

Pancakes with butter and maple syrup

Blueberries

Caffeine-free herb tea

Grape juice

Lunch

Egg salad sandwich

◆ Carrot salad

Ginger ale

Dinner

◆ Spaghetti with tomato-beef ragu

◆ Mixed salad greens with horseradish dressing

Vanilla pudding

DAY 3

Breakfast

Cereal (cornflakes, rice puffs, shredded wheat . . .) with milk

Mango

Caffeine-free herb tea

Apricot nectar

Lunch

Turkey sandwich

◆ Sliced tomatoes with vinaigrette dressing

Sparkling water

Dinner

Cheeseburger (with American cheese)

French fries

Homemade coleslaw

Strawberries with whipped cream

DAY 4

Salads & Crudités
Watch out for dressings made with vinegar (other than clear white vinegar) or with lemon juice. Use fresh (ideally homemade) as opposed to bottled dressings. Be careful about onions . . . although leeks, scallions, shallots and spring onions are okay. And stay away from adornments such as cheese and croutons, which tend to be MSG-rich. Tomatoes, too, can present a problem for some headache sufferers.

BROCCOLI	CHARD	LETTUCES OF ALL KINDS	PEPPERS
CABBAGE	CUCUMBERS		RADICCHIO
CARROTS	ENDIVE	MUSHROOMS	RADISHES
CAULIFLOWER	GARLIC	OLIVES	SPROUTS
CELERY	KALE	PARSLEY	TOMATOES

DAY 5

Breakfast

Waffles with butter and maple syrup

Cantaloupe

Caffeine-free herb tea

Pear juice

Lunch

Omelette

Buttered toast

Sliced cucumber seasoned with salt and pepper

Root beer (caffeine-free)

Dinner

♦ Pork tenderloin in curry sauce

Rice

♦ Mixed salad greens with vinaigrette dressing

Shortbread cookies

DAY 6

Breakfast

Buttered blueberry muffin

Apricots

Caffeine-free herb tea

Peach nectar

Lunch

♦ Mixed salad greens with grilled chicken and horseradish dressing

Crackers

Bottled water

Dinner

♦ Grilled sea bass with tomato salsa

Zucchini

Couscous

Mango sorbet

Vegetables & Starches

ARTICHOKES

ASPARAGUS

BAKED GOODS*

BEANS*

BEETS

BROCCOLI

BRUSSELS SPROUTS

CAULIFLOWER

CARROTS

CEREALS (NO RAISINS, NUTS OR CHOCOLATE)

CHICK PEAS (GARBANZOS)

CORN

COUSCOUS

FENNEL

MUSHROOMS

OKRA

PASTA

PEAS (NOT PODS)

PEPPERS

POLENTA

POTATOES

RICE (BEWARE OF SEASONED MIXTURES: MSG)

SQUASH

STRING BEANS

TURNIPS

YAMS

ZUCCHINI

*See Table 6, pages 74–75.

Breakfast

Soft- or hard-boiled egg

Buttered toast

Strawberries

Caffeine-free herb tea

Apple juice

Lunch

Grilled American cheese sandwich

Carrot sticks

Mixed berry juice

Dinner

◆ Roast chicken

Asparagus

Polenta (using plain polenta cornmeal)

◆ Vanilla ice cream with hot blueberry sauce

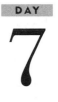

DAY

7

Snack Ideas

CAKES
(WITHOUT NUTS, CITRUS OR CHOCOLATE)

CARROT OR CELERY STICKS

COOKIES
(WITHOUT NUTS, RAISINS, PEANUT BUTTER OR CHOCOLATE)

COTTAGE CHEESE

CRACKERS
(SALTED, UNFLAVORED)

FRUITS*

GRANOLA (PLAIN)

ICE CREAM
(NO NUTS OR CHOCOLATE)

MELBA TOAST
(PLAIN)

OLIVES

POPCORN
(NO CHEESE OR OTHER FLAVORS)

POTATO CHIPS
(SALTED, UNFLAVORED)

PRETZELS (NOT FRESH-BAKED OR SOFT)

PUMPKIN SEEDS

SORBET
(NO CITRUS)

SUNFLOWER SEEDS

TOASTED CORN

TORTILLA CHIPS
(PLAIN)

VEGGIES*

*See Table 6, pages 74–75.

Recipes for Relief

Tomato Salsa*

(Makes 2 cups)

3 peeled tomatoes cut into small pieces

1 shallot

2 tablespoons chopped chives

1 tablespoon minced parsley

1 tablespoon tomato paste

2 tablespoons drained capers

2 tablespoons sliced black olives

Salt and pepper to taste

Mix all ingredients. Season with salt and pepper. Serve with grilled fish.

*Tomatoes may be triggers for some people.

Herb Salsa

(Makes 1 cup)

8 basil leaves

8 mint leaves

1/2 bunch parsley leaves

1 minced garlic clove

1 tablespoon Dijon mustard

1 tablespoon capers

2/3 cup olive oil

Salt and pepper to taste

Finely chop all ingredients in a blender or food processor. Serve at room temperature.

Vinaigrette Dressing

(Serves 2)

1/4 cup olive oil

1/2 teaspoon tarragon white wine vinegar

1/2 teaspoon Dijon mustard

1 tablespoon apple juice

Pinch of sugar

Salt and pepper to taste

Mix all ingredients well, preferably in a blender.

Horseradish Dressing*

(Makes 1 cup)

1/2 cup milk (2% or whole)

1 tablespoon heavy cream

1 tablespoon horseradish

1 tablespoon tomato paste

1 tablespoon minced fresh dill

Salt and pepper to taste

Blend all ingredients.

*Tomatoes may be triggers for some people.

Carrot Salad

(Serves 2)

2 shredded carrots

1 shredded apple

1 teaspoon vegetable oil

Salt, pepper and sugar to taste

Mix carrots and apple. Add oil, seasonings and sugar.

Tuna Salad

(Serves 2)

1 6-ounce can white tuna (drain well if packed in water or oil with hydrolyzed protein)

1 shredded carrot

1 chopped celery stalk

2 tablespoons sliced green olives

1 tablespoon capers

2 tablespoons mayonnaise

Salt and pepper to taste

Fluff tuna in mixing bowl. Add all other ingredients and mix well.

Crab Cakes

(Serves 2)

1 pound jumbo lump crabmeat

2 tablespoons bread crumbs (homemade with crunched dried bread)

$1/4$ cup mayonnaise

1 large egg

1 tablespoon minced parsley

Salt and pepper to taste

4 tablespoons melted butter

Combine all ingredients except butter and mix together. Form crab cakes and place on baking sheet; spoon melted butter over crab cakes. Broil for about 5 minutes, until lightly browned. Turn and broil for about 2 minutes more.

Roast Chicken

(Serves 4–6)

1 whole chicken (3–4 pounds)

Brine

2 quarts of water

$^1/_2$ cup salt

$^1/_2$ cup sugar

Stuffing

15–20 dried prunes (without sulfites)

1–2 peeled apples cut into eighths

2 coarsely chopped shallots

3 fresh thyme sprigs

Flavored butter

2 tablespoons softened unsalted butter

1 tablespoon fresh thyme, minced

1 tablespoon fresh ground pepper

1 tablespoon sweet paprika

In large container, dissolve salt and sugar in 2 quarts water; immerse chicken and refrigerate for at least 5 hours. Preheat oven to 425°. Remove chicken from container, rinse with cold water and pat dry. Mix prunes, apples and shallots; place inside chicken with thyme sprigs. Mix all ingredients for flavored butter in small bowl; apply all over chicken. Place chicken on rack and bake for 15 minutes. Reduce heat to 375°. Continue baking for about 1 hour or until chicken is crisp and deep golden brown, with 180° internal temperature of deep breast. Remove chicken from oven; let sit at room temperature for about 10 minutes. Carve and serve.

Tomato-Beef Ragu*

(Serves 4–6)

2 tablespoons olive oil

1 tablespoon butter

4 finely diced shallots

1 $^1/_2$ pounds ground beef

1 tablespoon minced fresh oregano, thyme, basil
  (or 1 teaspoon dry oregano, thyme, basil)

2 tablespoons minced fresh parsley

1 shredded carrot

1 chopped celery stalk

1 finely diced zucchini

1 15-ounce can peeled tomatoes cut into small pieces

1 12-ounce can tomato paste

Salt and pepper to taste

Heat oil and butter in skillet. Sauté shallots over medium heat for 3 minutes; add beef and brown well, stirring to separate clumps. Add herbs and vegetables, and cook for 3 minutes. Add tomatoes and tomato paste and season to taste. Let simmer for about 45 minutes. Serve over cooked spaghetti.

*Tomatoes may be triggers for some people.

Pork Tenderloin in Curry Sauce

(Serves 2)

2 tablespoons olive oil

1 tablespoon butter

1 diced shallot

1–2 mashed garlic cloves

1 pork tenderloin cut into 1" slices

1 yellow pepper cut into thin strips

1 zucchini cut into thin strips

1 cup thinly sliced mushrooms

1 tablespoon sweet curry

1 tablespoon hot curry

Salt and pepper to taste

$1/3$ cup water

$1/3$ cup heavy cream

Heat oil and butter in skillet. Sauté shallots and garlic for 3 minutes. Add pork; brown both sides. Add pepper, zucchini and mushroom. Cook for 3 minutes. Season with curry, salt and pepper. Add water and cream. Cook for 3 more minutes. Serve with rice.

Apricot Cake

(Serves 8)

$1/2$ stick unsalted butter

$1/2$ cup sugar

$1/2$ cup flour

$1/2$ teaspoon vanilla extract

Pinch of salt

3 egg yolks

1 whole egg

About 16 fresh apricots

Preheat oven to 350°. Butter and flour 10"-diameter spring-form pan. Beat butter and sugar until well blended; add egg yolks and whole egg and beat to blend. Mix in flour, vanilla extract and salt, and pour batter into prepared pan. Cut apricots into halves, remove pits and place on top of cake in single layer, cut side down. Bake for 45 minutes or until lightly brown. Serve at room temperature with vanilla ice cream.

Vanilla Ice Cream with Hot Blueberry Sauce

(Serves 8)

1 bag frozen blueberries

$1/4$ cup sugar

Pinch of cinnamon

1 quart vanilla ice cream

Dollop of whipped cream (optional)

Place defrosted berries in saucepan and heat over medium heat. Add sugar and cinnamon. Scoop ice cream into little bowls. Pour hot sauce over ice cream and serve immediately. Add whipped cream if desired.

Dietary Tips

REMEMBER, THE MIGRAINE-PREVENTIVE DIET is not a life sentence; it's a *tool* to help you control your headaches. The better you use it, the better it works. Once you've controlled your headaches, you can try to liberalize the diet. No one can follow the diet absolutely perfectly. *Just do the best you can.*

When you follow the diet, you'll find yourself eating healthier and feeling better in many ways, not just with fewer and milder headaches. For instance, if you're eager to lose weight, the diet can help. And by avoiding caffeine, you'll sleep better and have more energy. Don't be surprised if your heartburn (gastroesophageal reflux) improves, too.

The diet is just *part* of Step 2, which is just *one* step in the 1-2-3 Program. By itself, the diet may enable you to control your headaches as long as you're not rebounding (Step 1). If the diet alone doesn't work, address other aspects of Step 2 and move on to Step 3—*without backstepping.*

◆ Be prepared that caffeine withdrawal may stir up your headaches for a week or two. It might not, but be ready just in case, and *be tough*: it will have been well worth it once you get through it.

◆ Monosodium glutamate (MSG) is everywhere. Pay close attention to food labels, but don't forget that more often than not MSG is disguised under an alias (see Table 7, page 81). As much as possible, eat fresh foods—other than fresh *baked* goods.

◆ Although MSG is *out*, herbs and spices in general are *in*. Use them to make your food sing (but watch out for spice mixtures that contain MSG under one name or another).

◆ Surprisingly, aside from MSG (oddly considered "natural" by the FDA) and nitrites and nitrates as preservatives, most *artificial* ingredients used to preserve, color, texturize or otherwise enhance food products don't seem to be migraine triggers. Sulfites are an exception; they can be triggers when found in some wines, dried fruit and items at not-so-fresh salad bars.

- The diet is a special challenge when you eat in restaurants or at other people's homes. Just look out for the obvious culprits, find out what's been added that may be invisible and avoid what you can. There's a balance to be struck between reasonably protecting yourself and *not* driving everyone—waiters, family, friends and yourself—crazy.

- No protein shortage here. Help yourself to fresh meat and poultry, seafood of all kinds, eggs, milk, cream and cottage cheese, seeds and certain beans. Even if you choose to restrict certain items, such as meat, you should still be able to fulfill your nutritional requirements while following the migraine-preventive diet.

- If you live with someone, it's great if you can enlist his or her cooperation—especially when it comes to nixing the morning coffee!

- Learn from your mistakes. If you know you slipped up on the diet and you get a headache . . . well, don't miss the point. And even if you're not aware of cutting corners, look back at the past day or two's intake when a headache strikes for no other apparent reason.

Up, Up and Away

Sometimes it helps to plan ahead. I have patients who bring their own food to nibble in airports or on planes, because otherwise it's awfully tough to avoid dietary triggers in those settings.

News flash: If you think you'd be wise to accept the flight attendant's offer of the salty snack mix rather than the alternative choice, headache-inducing peanuts, think again. That mix is *loaded* with MSG. You'd really be wise to avoid both and bring something of your own—something safe.

And the next time you fly I hope you'll think of me and smile as you gaze down upon the food tray you're served, on which sits—both out in the open and under cover—one dietary trigger after another. *Better idea:* Next time, bag it. ◆

Once you've controlled your headaches—and maintained control for *at least* four months—you can decide if you want to try rocking your boat by reintroducing potential triggers. If you do so, keep these points in mind:

- *Don't* add back caffeine—but you can try decaf coffee or tea.
- The list of dietary triggers in Table 6 (pages 74–75) is roughly prioritized by potency, but since everyone's different, your biggest problem might be an item at the bottom of the list.
- Try first adding back the items you most crave.
- Don't try adding back items you don't really care about. (Why would you? It's not worth it.)
- Keep an eye out for a day or two after cheating on the diet—the triggering effect may be delayed that long.
- Don't forget that your tolerance of a dietary trigger will vary from day to day, depending on your level of other (background) triggers. Getting away with a reintroduced dietary trigger one day doesn't mean it won't be a trigger on another.
- Your tolerance of a dietary trigger may also vary based on time of day. You might be able to get away with alcohol or chocolate in the evening without a headache even on the next day, but not if you indulge earlier in the day.
- The more of a dietary trigger you consume, the more likely you'll suffer. The same goes for combining multiple triggers within a day or two: the greater the quantity, the greater the risk.
- When reintroducing additional cheeses, you might best tolerate younger varieties: fresh goat or mozzarella, mascarpone or provolone, for example.
- Being able to cook with lemon or lime juice, white wine or onions makes life a lot easier, and you can try adding these back . . . but *carefully*, one at a time.
- Ditto for regular vinegar—in addition to the clear white versions allowable initially—and lemon juice in homemade salad dressings.

- If you drink alcohol, you're most likely to get away with vodka or white wine.
- If you choose to cheat on the diet (by bingeing on chocolate once in a while, for example) and you suffer a headache as a result, that's okay . . . *you still have control.*
- In the long run, the diet is flexible: you can adjust your compliance according to need, as other triggers—and consequently your headaches and other migraine symptoms—rise and fall.

Index

Page numbers in italics indicate sidebar text.

C

N

T

About the Author

DAVID BUCHHOLZ GRADUATED from the University of Pennsylvania School of Medicine and for 14 years served as director of the Neurological Consultation Clinic at Johns Hopkins, where he remains an associate professor. He has published more than 150 scientific publications and has given over 450 invited lectures nationally and internationally.

Aside from helping headache sufferers, Dr. Buchholz enjoys spending time with his wife and three children at home in Baltimore. His other interests include working in his garden, traveling and trying to stay fit.